Excel™ for Clinical Governance

Alan Gillies

Professor in Information Management
University of Central Lancashire

T0186284

Radcliffe Medical Press

© 2001 Alan Gillies

Radcliffe Medical Press Ltd
18 Marcham Road, Abingdon, Oxon OX14 1AA

All rights reserved. No part of this publication may be reproduced, stored in a retrieval system or transmitted, in any form or by any means, electronic, mechanical, photocopying, recording or otherwise without the prior permission of the copyright owner.

British Library Cataloguing in Publication Data

A catalogue record for this book is available from the British Library.

ISBN 1 85775 468 9

Typeset by Action Publishing Technology, Gloucester
Printed and bound by TJ International Ltd, Padstow, Cornwall

Contents

Preface

This book has been designed to help all healthcare professionals trying to implement clinical governance. It is based upon the belief that in order to make clinical governance work, it is necessary to have good quality information and be able to manage it effectively. The book provides a series of governance scenarios drawn from a range of healthcare situations – they're supposed to make you feel at home.

As with most of my books, it tries to do at least six impossible things:

1 Talk about information in an interesting way.
2 Show how computers can actually be useful.
3 Explain how to get you to love statistics.
4 Make clinical governance work.
5 Improve the quality of patient care.
6 Make you smile while reading a book about governance.

The book assumes a basic knowledge of computers and Windows95™ or Windows98™. The book does not assume any prior knowledge of Excel2000™. A typical reader might have used computers for word processing or used a clinical system.

The book assumes that you the reader are a healthcare professional, probably based in the NHS. However, the scenarios are also relevant to private healthcare and the occupational health sector.

Each section starts with a description of the scenario, and a list of the tasks and Excel™ functions covered within that section. Each concludes with a set of exercises designed to reinforce the learning outcomes from that scenario.

Crucially, the book includes an appendix on how to extract data from the closed proprietary systems so often found in the NHS. This deals in detail with systems from primary care. However, general principles are also given for other sectors and systems.

There is a website associated with this book at:
www.primarycareonline.co.uk/imit/excel.

While it will be advantageous to have access to this, the book is designed to be largely accessible without web access. For example, where possible, alternative sources are given for every resource identified as being available over the web.

An accompanying CD is also available which provides access to data sheets. It also has other resources, particularly ScreenCam Movies which provide model answers for the scenarios.

The book is based upon Windows98™ and Excel2000™. Users of Windows95™ will notice little, if any, difference. Users of Excel™ for Windows95™ or Excel97™ should also notice little difference. For a full discussion of these issues see the website. Non-surfing readers, please contact the author for more information.

The book was fun to write. I hope it's fun to read.

Alan Gillies
October 2000

professor@alangillies.co.uk

How to use the book

The book is organised into a series of scenarios. Broadly speaking, it is probably best if you read them in order. However, you may well find some material surplus to requirements. In particular, the *Before we start* section will be old hat to some readers.

There are a number of common elements that recur throughout the book. At the start of each chapter there is an **In this chapter** box which includes details of the tasks covered and the Excel functions covered for the first time. The different points are distinguished by their respective bullets:

In this chapter

This chapter will tell you:

• what tasks the chapter covers

 what Excel functions are covered

Each **governance scenario** is described at the start of the section:

Governance scenario I

Each scenario ends with **exercises** that are designed to reinforce the learning outcomes from that section:

Exercise

The answers to the exercises are found on the website, as are any data sheets required within the chapters. For non-surfers, an accompanying CD is available which also includes extra resources such as ScreenCam Movies.

The text contains practical hints to help you – these are shown by the **Hint** icon and a box:

Hint

Web references in the text are indicated by a web icon within a box:

Other features of the text are **think boxes** which raise issues for further thought. They are designed for discussion, and would really benefit from the chance to discuss the answers with colleagues, either in a group situation or in a series of one-to-one encounters.

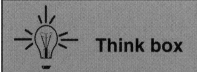

Principles of good practice are key practical issues. They represent an action that is good or best practice.

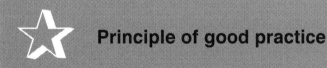

Health warnings are provided as messages to prevent common errors or confusion:

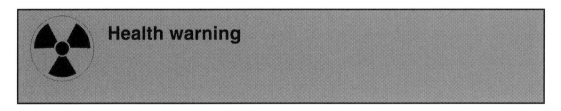

In order to make your life easier instructions in the text are bulleted and distinguished as either mouse or keyboard actions:

⌨   This is a keyboard action.

🖱   This is a mouse action.

Before we start

In this chapter

This chapter will tell you:

• more about conventions used in this book

• about your computer

• about Windows95 and Windows98

 what Excel2000 looks like

 how to move around in Excel

 how to identify or 'highlight' areas of the sheet

OK, so this is the bit that everyone misses out. I know that. All I ask is that you read the first bit. After that, if you know your way around Windows and Excel you can skip the introduction, but please read the bit at the end of the chapter where I deal with some more conventions used in the book. We shall begin with a few health warnings.

Health warning

This is not a statistics book. It is not even written by someone who claims to be a statistician. All I offer is that I know what I don't know, and that I gave the text to a statistician to read and remove the gravest errors.

The moral is, if you are going to use any of the more complex stuff in anger, go and talk to a statistician. Failing that go and read a real statistics book such as *Practical Statistics for Medical Research* by Douglas Altman, and then go and find a statistician to explain the bits you don't understand.

I have tried to ensure that this book is relatively rigorous and also simple to understand. This is clearly impossible, or in statistical terms very, very improbable!

To get started, we will introduce Windows, and for those still reading against your better judgement, thank you. If you know all about Windows, skip to the end of this chapter for the summary of the conventions used in the book to represent mouse and keyboard actions in the main text.

An introduction to Windows

Windows is the system that brought computers to the masses. Odd really, because when it was first introduced in 1990, it was neither new (the idea was at least 15 years old), the best around (everyone said that the Apple system was better) or in the early days, even particularly reliable. However, it has made Bill Gates the richest man in the world, so it must do something right!

Windows uses what is known as WIMPs: windows, icons, mice and pointers. The screen is supposed to represent a desktop. Work currently on the desktop is displayed in windows which can be re-arranged on the desktop in much the same way as papers and files can be re-arranged on a desk. Items not currently open on the desktop may be shown as icons. These are small images that indicate the availability of items and display their type by the particular item in use.

An essential item for ease of use is a graphical user interface (known as a GUI, for those who need polite conversation at a computer geek's cocktail party). In the Windows environment this is the mouse, which can drive a variety of pointers (principally arrows and crosses) around the screen. The use of the mouse and the associated screen pointer also facilitates the selection of items from pop-up and pull-down menus.

The most important feature of Windows is its standardisation. This means that almost all Windows applications work in the same way. This considerably reduces learning time for any one application and allows one to 'guess' how many of the operations in an application might work from the experience of another. Crucially for us, if you are already familiar with Word then many of the operations in Excel will, in part, already be familiar to you. For example, using Cut and Paste in Edit is the same in Excel and Word. It also means that, if you are using an application for the first time then, having followed this text, you should be well on the way to understanding other Windows applications.

The next section provides an introduction to the Windows environment.

Finding Excel in Windows

Most computers when switched on produce an opening screen that looks something like this:

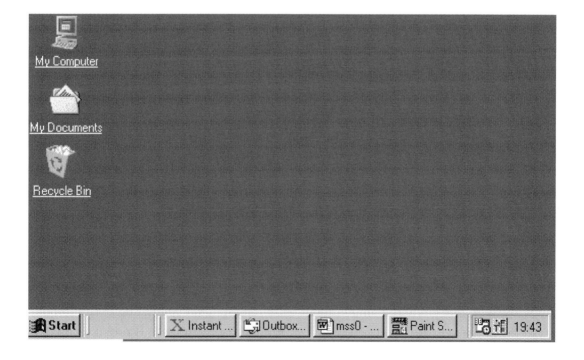

To start:

🖑 **Click** on ▨Start.

The Start menu should appear.

From this menu:

🖑 **Click** on Programs.

From this menu:

🖑 **Click** on Microsoft Office.

From this menu:

🖑 **Click** on Microsoft Excel.

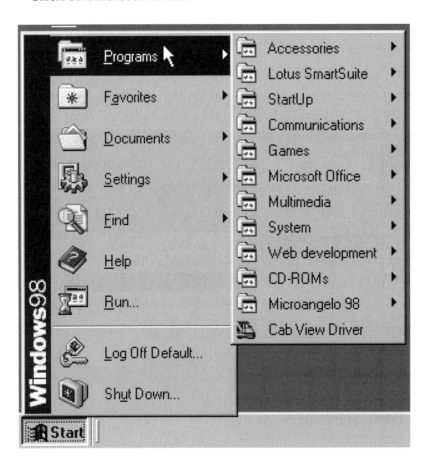

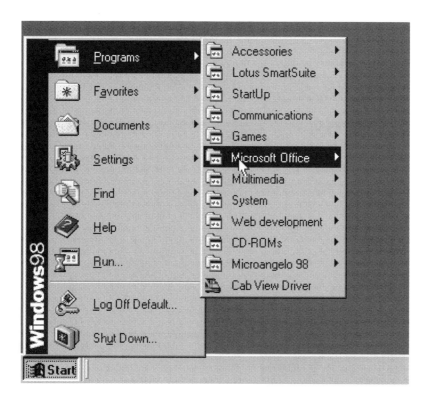

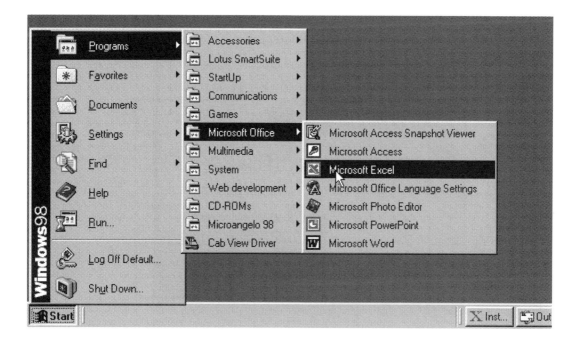

For those who want to know more about Windows, there are some excel-lent texts around such as *Windows98 for Dummies*. Do not be put off by the title or the bright yellow cover. This kind of book can be really helpful.

For us, we shall consider the opening Excel screen. It should look something like this:

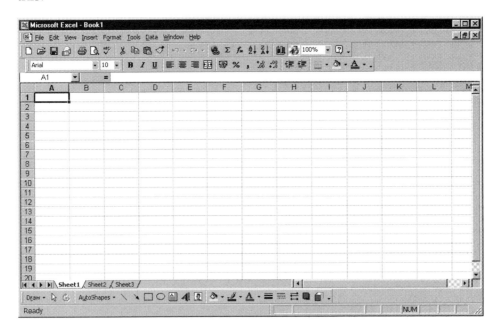

Excel is a spreadsheet. Essentially, a spreadsheet is an electronic piece of paper divided into rows and columns. The intersection of a row and column forms a cell.

Each cell is identified by the row and column that it occupies:

	A	B	C
1	cell A1	cell B1	cell C1
2	cell A2	cell B2	cell C2
3	cell A3	cell B3	cell C3

Schematic representation of rows, columns and cells.

Unlike a piece of paper, each cell can contain more than just text or a number; most importantly, it can contain a formula detailing how the value displayed in that cell is calculated.

Excel operates in the Windows environment making full use of windows, icons, the mouse and pointers. It is controlled largely by using the mouse to point at objects and 'clicking' the mouse to activate the object, rather than typing in commands.

Excel uses a lot of toolbars. These are a set of 'buttons' which, when clicked on, perform an operation. They provide shortcuts to a number of standard operations covering functions such as drawing, macros, charting and so on.

Toolbars

At this stage we shall start with the main toolbar. The toolbar buttons in the upper row, from left to right are:

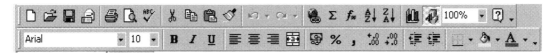

- New workbook
- Open workbook
- Save workbook
- Email
- Print
- Print preview
- Spell checker
- Cut
- Copy
- Paste
- Format painter
- Undo
- Redo
- Insert hyperLink
- Internet
- Autosum
- Autofunction
- Sort (ascending)
- Sort (descending)
- Chart wizard
- Drawing

- Zoom
- Help.

The second row is known as the formatting toolbar, and includes, from left to right, buttons for:

- Font
- Font size
- Bold
- Italic
- Underline
- Left align
- Centre align
- Right align
- Align across multiple cells
- Currency
- Percentage
- Comma style
- Increase decimal
- Decrease decimal
- Decrease indent
- Increase indent
- Borders
- Fill colour
- Text colour.

Rather than give you indigestion at this point, we shall delay explanation of each function until later in the text. The toolbar is simply a shortcut way of entering commands into the computer.

For example:

🖱 **Click** on the 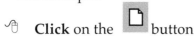 button

🖱 **Select** 'File' from the menu bar

🖱 **Select** 'New' from the 'File' menu.

In fact, the above is just one of several toolbars which are designed to help us use Excel more quickly and easily. In what follows we shall make use of the toolbars as much as possible.

If you're not sure which button does what, then simply move the mouse so that the pointer on the screen lies over the required toolbar button. After a short pause, a message will appear:

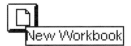

Movement around the sheet

Vertical and horizontal movement works as for any other application. Place the arrow in the scroll bar and click on the square down arrow screen button to achieve single cell movement, or hold down for multi-cell movement. To move selectively up or down (right or left), hold the left mouse button down on the scroll bar button (i.e. the blank button which is situated within the scroll bar) and drag it gently down the bar (or rightward along the bar). Notice the highlight (the faint square outline) move. When the mouse button is released the scroll button will move to the highlight and movement in the spreadsheet will be effected.

Highlighting areas of the sheet

Highlighting areas of the sheet is a fundamental operation that will allow us to copy, move, format or otherwise edit areas of the sheet.

Take the blank sheet on the screen in front of you:

🖰 Place the arrow in cell B3, hold down the left-hand button and 'drag' the mouse across the sheet to cell F8.

Hint

Please note that later in the text, we shall simply record this instruction as:

🖰 **Highlight** B3 to F8.

The end result of highlighting this region of the sheet is shown below.
 To extend the highlighted area:

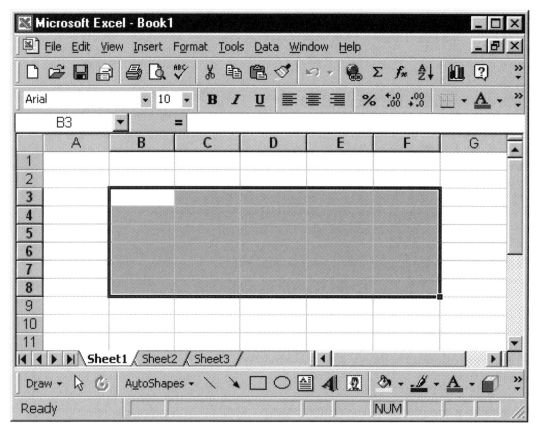 **Hold** down the [⇧] key and **hold** down the left mouse button simultaneously and **drag** the mouse across the tabletop to cell H8 and release.

There should now be a highlighted area extending from B3 down to H8.

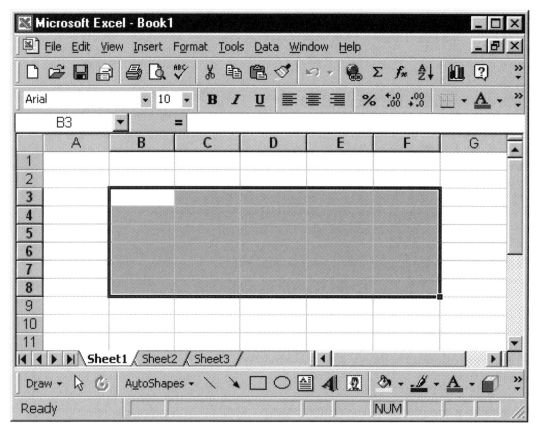

Empty sheet with highlighted area from B3 to F8.

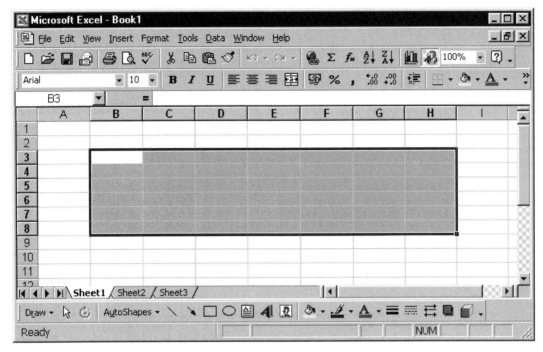

Highlighted area extended to H8.

Alternatively, you may wish to highlight two or more separate areas. This commonly occurs when you want to select data together with labels. For example, to highlight the areas B3 to F3 and B5 to F8:

Highlight the cells B3 to F3, as above

Hold down the [Ctrl] key and **click** on B5

Hold down the left mouse button simultaneously, and

Drag the mouse across the tabletop to cell F8 and release.

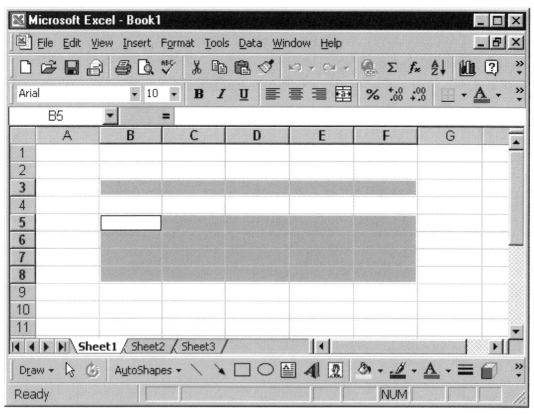

There should now be two highlighted areas extending from B3 to F3 and down from B5 to F8.

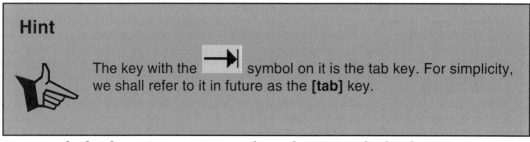

Hint

The key with the ──▶│ symbol on it is the tab key. For simplicity, we shall refer to it in future as the **[tab]** key.

Pressing the [tab] or ↵ key moves you through cells in a highlighted area:

⌨ **Press** [tab] for horizontal movement

⌨ **Press** ↵ for vertical movement.

You can highlight the entire sheet by selecting the square grey button at the top left-hand corner of the sheet:

🖰 **Click** on 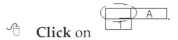 .

Using more than one sheet in a book

At the bottom of the sheet is a set of tabs:

The tabs displayed at the bottom of the sheet.

The sheet you see is simply the first of a large number available to you. A typical use of this facility might involve annual data on prescribing costs. On the top sheet one would have data relating to the current year. On the sheets beneath, one could have data from previous years. This would allow comparison over time. This facility is often referred to as using multidimensional spreadsheets. In such a case, time becomes the third dimension:

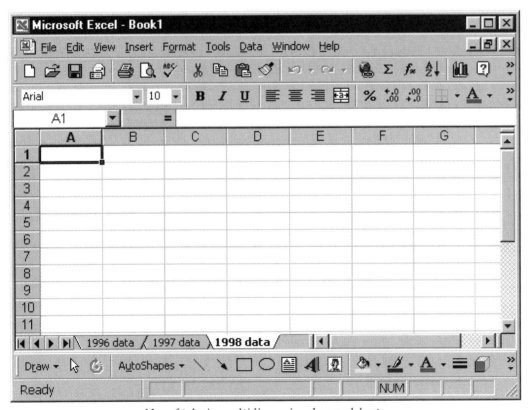

Use of tabs in multidimensional spreadsheets.

Exercise

 Click on each of the menus in turn to familiarise yourself with what's there. By the time you get to the end of the book, hopefully you'll know what most options do.

Summary of mouse and keyboard action conventions used in this book

Mouse action	Explanation
Move	Requires you to move the whole mouse around physically on the desk. The action is mimicked on the screen.
Click	Requires you to press once on the left-hand button of the mouse to highlight a specific object or cell.
Right-click	Requires you to press once on the right-hand button of the mouse to highlight a specific object or cell.
Double-click	Requires you to press twice in quick succession (almost like an involuntary twitch!) on the left-hand button of the mouse without moving the mouse in between.
Drag	Requires you to move to an object, press down the left-hand button of the mouse and without releasing the button, move the mouse to the location required on the screen. Once at the destination, release the mouse button. This operation is used to 'highlight' areas in Excel see next entry.
Highlight	Requires you to highlight a range of cells by dragging the mouse over the required range.

Keyboard action	Explanation
Type	Requires you to type whatever follows.
Press	Requires you to press a single key or in some cases a combination of keys.

My first governance exercise with Excel

In this chapter

This chapter will tell you how to:

- monitor levels of attendance at a health promotion clinic

- manage basic data required for the above

- present results in graphical form

enter data into an Excel sheet

copy and move data within the sheet

use the AutoFill to copy formulae and save work

use pre-defined functions, and the Autosum facility

format: data types, fonts, presentation

save and print the sheet

produce simple graphs.

Introduction

The Sony Corporation has brought us much: the Walkman, the Trinitron television tube. But one of their neatest ideas is the *My First Sony* concept.

My First Sony is a range of toys aimed at introducing the young potential Sony consumer to the company. As such, they are toy versions of adult products that allow the user to familiarise themselves with the basic concepts.

This first governance scenario is simplified to provide a way of introducing basic concepts. The scenarios which follow are more realistic, but necessarily more complex.

So here it is – my first governance exercise with Excel – with apologies to the Sony Corporation of Japan.

The scenario

A practice has introduced a well-woman clinic. During the first year of operation, the level of activity has been monitored to assist in resource management and to investigate how many of the target population of 2000 women have used the facility within a 12 month period.

Getting started: opening a sheet

When you first open Excel, you get a blank workbook on the screen.

The attendance data for the well-woman clinic is shown below:

1998	Attendees
Jan	52
Feb	71
Mar	96
Apr	124
May	150
Jun	168
Jul	117
Aug	78
Sep	121
Oct	134
Nov	152
Dec	117

First, we enter this data into our blank sheet. In our new sheet, cell A1 will be highlighted, so we can start typing straight away:

⌨ **Type** 1998

⌨ **Press** [tab] to move to B1.

Hint

 The [tab] key is a really convenient way to move between cells.

Remember: ↵ enters text and moves down a cell; [tab] enters text and moves to the right.

At cell B1:

⌨ **Type** Attendees

🖱 **Click** on A2

⌨ **Type** Jan

⌨ **Press** [tab] to B1

⌨ **Type** 52

🖱 **Click** on cell A3

⌨ **Type** Feb

⌨ **Press** [tab] to move to B1

⌨ **Type** 71

🖱 **Click** on A4

⌨ **Type** Mar

⌨ **Press** [tab] to move to cell B1

⌨ **Type** 96.

And so on, until it looks like the one I prepared earlier, shown below:

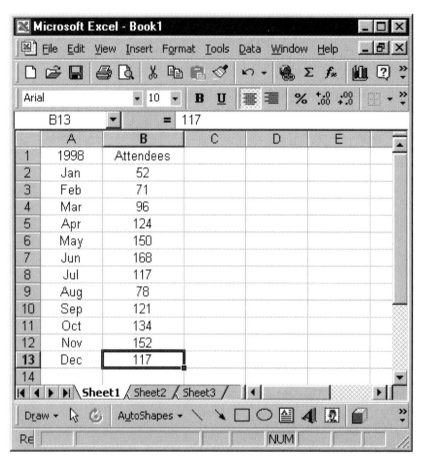

And there you have it – My first Excel sheet.

The first thing we'll do is to save your handiwork. There are nearly always at least two ways to do things in Excel. For example, to save the file we could either:

🖱 **Click** on 🖫 in the toolbar

or

🖱 **Click** on File in the menu toolbar

🖱 **Click** on Save on the File menu
or

⌨ **Hold down** [Ctrl] and **Press** S.

Either way, you end up at the Save As dialog box:

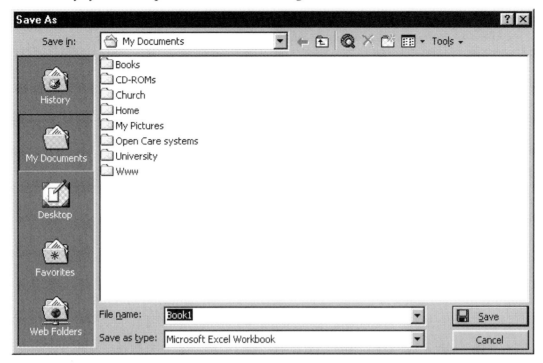

Hint

A dialog box is a box that allows you to enter into a dialogue with the computer. The spelling is American, or as the *OED* puts it 'computer usage'.

Hint

It is a general principle in Excel that the toolbars provide a quick method but using the menus gives maximum flexibility. The keyboard shortcuts are even quicker than the toolbars but require you to remember the relevant key combinations.

However, there is no correct way to do things – you choose.

Type a name for your sheet. It will replace the highlighted text:

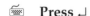 **Type** My first Excel spreadsheet.

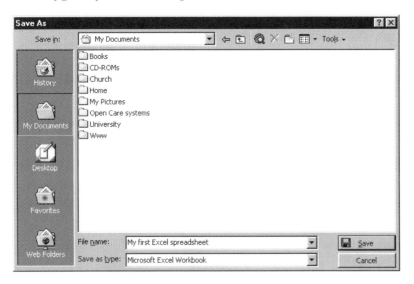

 Click on [▣ Save]

or

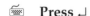 **Press** ↵

⭐ ## Principle of good practice

It is a good idea to save your work regularly in case of accidents. Also ensure that the automatic recovery facility is switched on and set up to save your work frequently.

If your Tools menu doesn't include an Autosave option, then look up AutoSave in the Help facility:

- **Click** on Help in the menu bar
- **Click** on Contents and Index
- **Click** on the Index tab
- **Type** Autosave
- **Click** on Display.

YOU HAVE BEEN WARNED!

Now that the sheet has been saved, let's close it down. This demonstrates more about Excel. It also allows you to go off and have a cup of coffee should you wish to.

To close the sheet, either:

🖰 **Click** on ☒ at the top right-hand corner of the sheet

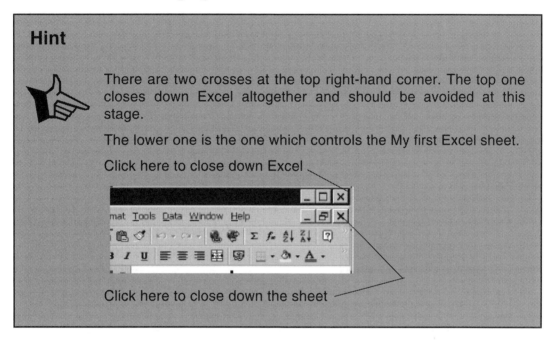

Hint

There are two crosses at the top right-hand corner. The top one closes down Excel altogether and should be avoided at this stage.

The lower one is the one which controls the My first Excel sheet.

Click here to close down Excel

Click here to close down the sheet

or

🖰 **Click** on <u>F</u>ile in the menu toolbar

🖰 **Click** on <u>C</u>lose on the File menu.

To return to the sheet, we need to open it:

🖰 **Click** on 📂

or

🖰 **Click** on <u>F</u>ile in the menu toolbar

🖰 **Click** on <u>O</u>pen on the File menu

🖰 **Click** on ☐ OK ☐ to open the workbook.

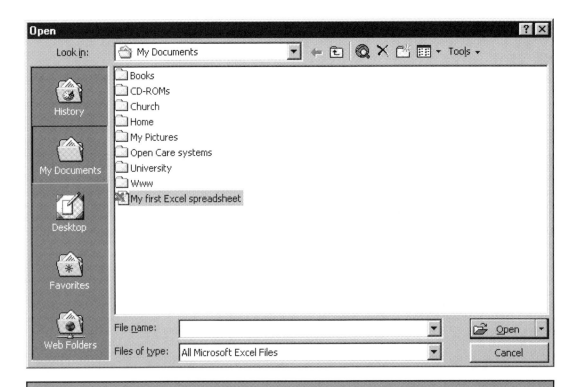

Hint

The File menu is where you can do all your file management, including opening, closing, saving and printing your worksheet files. One of the most useful bits is the list of recently used files at the bottom of the File menu. Otherwise, the main functions are duplicated on the first five toolbar buttons:

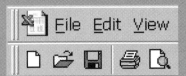

These buttons correspond to New, Open, Save, Print and Print preview.

Where keyboard shortcuts exist they are shown on the menu, e.g. Ctrl+N for New.

Hint

It is generally good practice to store files in different directories, using a different directory for each project.

Remember, however, that if you store your files in different directories, you may need to select from the directory box or drive box if the file you require is not in the current directory or drive. You may also have to slide down the scroll bar if the file you require is not currently showing in the file selection box.

Our sheet is now back with us – we will start to refine it.

First, we need to enter a title for our sheet. To do this we insert an extra row at the top of the sheet:

🖰 **Click** on A1

🖰 **Click** on Insert in the menu bar

🖰 **Click** on Rows on the insert menu

⌨ **Type** Planned and actual activity at the Well-Woman Clinic 1998

⌨ **Press** ↵ .

Hint

Do not be concerned about the title flooding over into adjacent cells. The text is all stored in A1.

The figures for planned activity are as follows:

1998	Planned
Jan	50
Feb	75
Mar	100
Apr	100
May	125
Jun	125
Jul	125
Aug	125
Sep	125
Oct	125
Nov	125
Dec	125

Exercise

Enter the data in Column C and change the headings so that the sheet appears as below. Refer back to putting in the original data if you're stuck.

See the final result below.

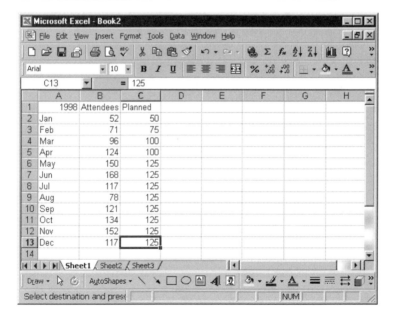

Formulae

Now we will enter our first formula. This is important, because this is where the computer starts to do the work. The art of using a spreadsheet is constructive laziness: never do yourself what the computer can do for you!

First of all we calculate the size of the over or under-utilisation for each month:

🖰 **Click** on D2

⌨ **Type** (Over)utilisation

⌨ **Type** = B3-C3

All formulae begin with = in Excel. This tells it to calculate something.

⌨ **Press** ↵.

This puts 2 in D3, the difference between the actual use (B3) and the planned use (C3).

Hint

If you are worried about typing errors then mistakes are easily corrected:

🖰 **Double-click** on cell containing incorrect text (B3 in this case)

🖰 **Move** the I-bar pointer to the immediate right of the error

🖰 **Click** (note that another flashing bar I appears within the text).

If incorrectly placed the flashing bar can be moved using keyboard arrow keys:

⌨ Use ← & [Del] keys to remove characters to the left or right of I flashing bar respectively

⌨ To insert characters just type them in

⌨ Press ↵ to end edit or Press [Esc] to end edit and retain the original text.

We now repeat this for each month but at this point we need to invoke my principle of constructive laziness:

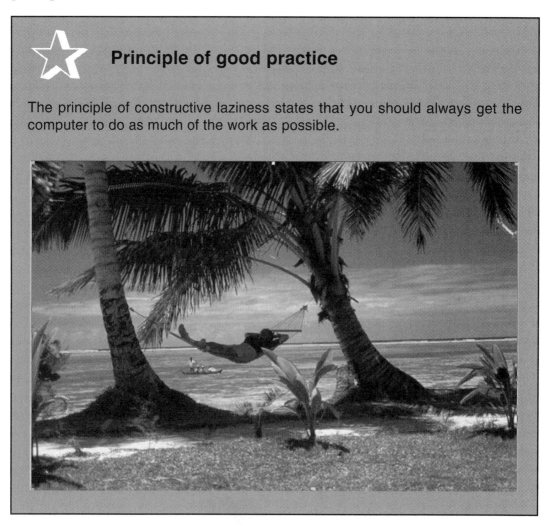

⭐ Principle of good practice

The principle of constructive laziness states that you should always get the computer to do as much of the work as possible.

Spreadsheets offer us a facility to copy formulae down a column or across a row. As they move down or across, they change to take account of their new position. Thus, if we copy our formula down the column, Excel will calculate:

=B4-C4 in D4

=B5-C5 in D5

=B6-C6 in D6

etc.

Hint

For the record, and so that you can show off to your friends in trendy wine bars, this is known as *relative referencing*. More importantly, sometimes you need to know how to switch it off and keep formula the same as you copy them across or down. We will use this in the next scenario.

To copy the formula down the column:

 Click on D3.

Note that in the bottom right-hand corner of the highlighted cell there is a little black square which changes to a small black cross as the cursor moves over it:

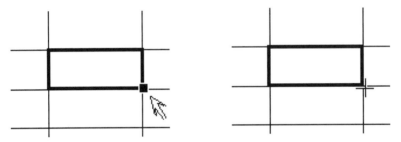

Drag the little black square down as far as D14.

If the cross is dragged to the right we can outline a row from B10 to M10. As the mouse is dragged down the cells are marked with a grey outline. When the mouse is released, the formulae are copied down:

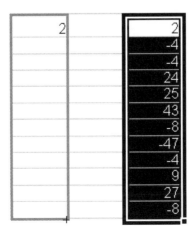

 Move the pointer away and **click** on another cell to remove the highlighting.

The sheet should now look like the one below:

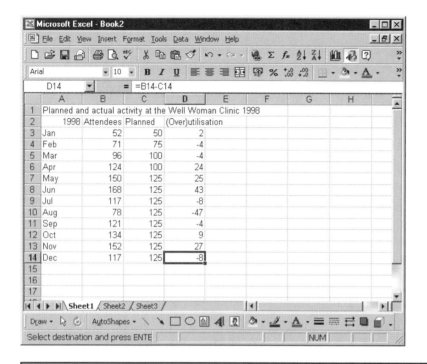

Hint

This is Excel's **AutoFill** function that is easy to use and of which more will be heard later.

In future, the text will simply say:

🖱 **AutoFill** down from D3 to D14

for the operation just completed.

Health warning

AutoFill is not always appropriate for your calculations. Always check them carefully to make sure that Excel did what you wanted by looking at the formulae on the edit line.

There is an alternative method using the menus. To use it we must first undo our **AutoFill** command:

🖱 **Click** on ↺ to undo the last action (one to remember!)

🖱 **Highlight** D3 down to D14

🖱 **Click** on Edit in the menu bar

🖱 **Click** on Fill on the Edit menu

🖱 **Click** on Down in the sub-menu

🖱 **Move** the pointer away and **click** on another cell to remove the highlighting.

The result should be the same.

Many formulae use predefined functions built into Excel, again fulfilling our principle of constructive laziness. Most require us to do some work, and we leave these to the next scenario, but the **AutoSum** feature is so simple we introduce it now.

First, let's add another label to our sheet:

🖱 **Click** on A15

⌨ **Type** TOTAL ⏎

🖱 **Highlight** B15 to D15

🖱 **Click** on Σ on the toolbar.

Excel adds each column and puts the total in the highlighted cell. Note that it can handle more than one column at once. This is Excel's **AutoSum** and it can be used at the end of rows.

Moving around the spreadsheet

Hint

To return to the top left-hand corner of the sheet at any time:

⌨ **Press** [Ctrl] and [Home] together.

We have already seen that it is easy to move around the spreadsheet using the scroll bars. In a large sheet it can be quite tedious to do this if you know that you want to alter information in one particular cell. To move to a specific cell:

🖰 **Click** on <u>E</u>dit from the menu bar

🖰 **Click** on <u>G</u>o To

or alternatively,

⌨ **Press** [F5].

Either should bring the Go To dialog box onto the screen.

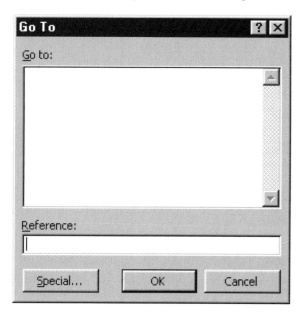

⌨ **Type** A3↵

🖰 **Click** on OK .

Improving presentation

Column D is too narrow for the label (Over)utilisation. We can change its width by using the mouse:

🖰 **Move** the cursor to column label D at the top of the first column

🖰 **Move** to right-hand side of cell between Column D and Column E.

Note that the cross pointer changes to an iron cross.

🖰 **Drag** the iron cross cursor to the right.

A faint vertical grey line appears below the cross as the mouse moves to the right. The column will widen when you release the button.

🖰 A second way to change the column width is to place the cursor as above, but to **double-click** instead of dragging. This will perform a best fit to accommodate the entries in the column.

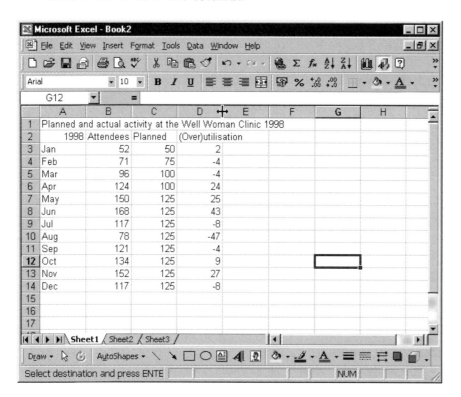

	A	B	C	D	E	F	G	H
1	Planned and actual activity at the Well Woman Clinic 1998							
2	1998	Attendees	Planned	(Over)utilisation				
3	Jan	52	50	2				
4	Feb	71	75	-4				
5	Mar	96	100	-4				
6	Apr	124	100	24				
7	May	150	125	25				
8	Jun	168	125	43				
9	Jul	117	125	-8				
10	Aug	78	125	-47				
11	Sep	121	125	-4				
12	Oct	134	125	9				
13	Nov	152	125	27				
14	Dec	117	125	-8				
15								
16								
17								

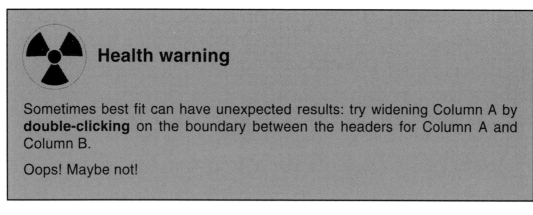

Health warning

Sometimes best fit can have unexpected results: try widening Column A by **double-clicking** on the boundary between the headers for Column A and Column B.

Oops! Maybe not!

Undo this action:

🖱 **Click** on ↶.

As usual, there is a further range of options available from the menus. To find them:

🖱 **Click** on Format in the menu bar

🖱 **Click** on Column in the Format menu

🖱 **Click** on Width in the sub-menu.

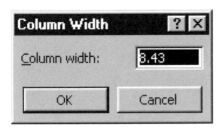

🖱 **Click** on Cancel.

This option is useful when you want to set a number of columns to the same width. For example:

🖱 **Click** on the header for Column A

🖱 **Drag** across as far as Column D, selecting Columns A to D

🖱 **Click** on Format in the menu bar

🖱 **Click** on Column in the Format menu

🖱 **Click** on Width in the sub-menu

⌨ **Type** 10 as the column width

🖱 **Click** on OK.

Formatting text

We can change many other aspects of presentation either from the tool bars or from a shortcut menu or from the Format menu. Most of the formatting option toolbar buttons appear on the formatting toolbar below the main toolbar. From left to right, these are:

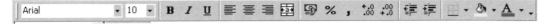

- Font (typeface)
- Font size
- Bold
- Italic
- Underline
- Left align
- Centre align
- Right align
- Centre across multiple cells
- Currency format
- Percentage format
- Comma delimiters
- Increase decimal
- Decrease decimal
- Reduce indent
- Increase indent
- Borders
- Shading
- Font colour.

One of the simplest formatting operations is the alignment of text. Text may be left- right- or centre-aligned. To illustrate this:

- **Highlight** Column A in our sheet
- **Click** on ▤ to left align the cells
- **Highlight** Columns B to D
- **Click** on ▤ to centre align the cells.

The result is shown below:

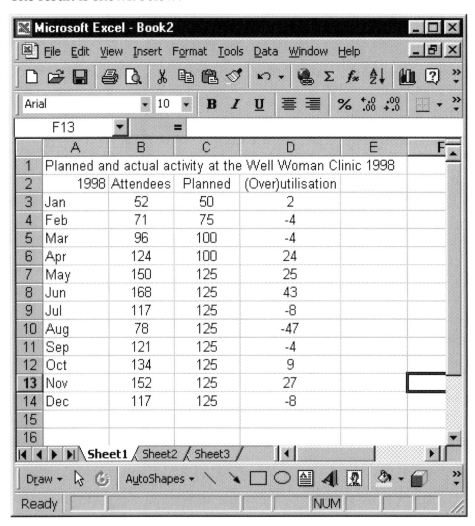

An alternative approach is to access the Format Cells dialog box. As always, the menus offer even more options. To access the Format Cells dialog box to see what's available:

🖱 **Click** on Format in the menu bar

🖱 **Click** on Cells in the Format menu.

There are untold riches here. For example, if we:

🖰 **Click** on the Alignment tab, the following dialog box appears:

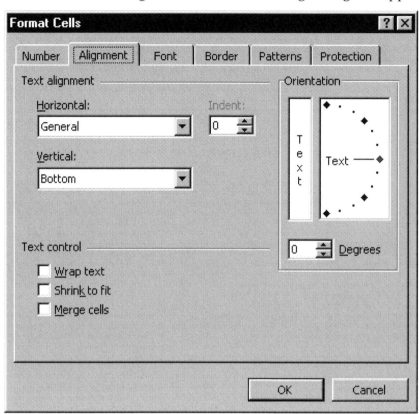

We can align the text in the vertical and horizontal directions or even rotate it through any angle between +90° and –90°.

🖰 **Click** on [Cancel] when you've had your fill of Aladdin's cave.

The other major formatting option available for text is the style of text. This can be achieved from the toolbar.

To change our headings to *italics*, highlight the range A2 to D2, then:

🖰 **Click** on *I*.

If we repeat the action, the italics are removed:

🖰 **Click** on *I*.

To **embolden** the text,

🖰 **Click** on **B**.

Now if we italicise the text, we get both bold and italics:

🖑 **Click** on *I* .

The titles should now look like:

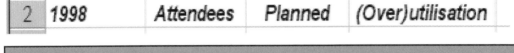

Or when the highlighting is removed by clicking somewhere else and Column D widened to do it justice:

Hint

The same result can be achieved from the keyboard. With a range of cells highlighted:

⌨ **Press** [Ctrl] and B together to embolden

⌨ **Press** [Ctrl] and I together to italicise.

We can change the font size using the drop down box containing the point size located near to the font display.

Try it on the overall title:

🖑 **Click** on A1

🖑 **Click** on ▾ next to the point size box

🖑 **Select** 12 from the drop down list.

The font may also be changed from the drop down list. The current font name is Arial.

To change the entire table to Times New Roman:

🖑 **Highlight** A1 to D15

🖑 **Click** on ▾ next to the font name box

🖑 **Select** Times New Roman from the drop down list.

All these options and more can be accessed from the Font tab in the Format cells dialog box. To examine these options and with the cells still highlighted:

🖰 **Click** on Format in the menu bar

🖰 **Click** on Cells in the Format menu

🖰 **Click** on the Font tab.

Another treasure trove of goodies!

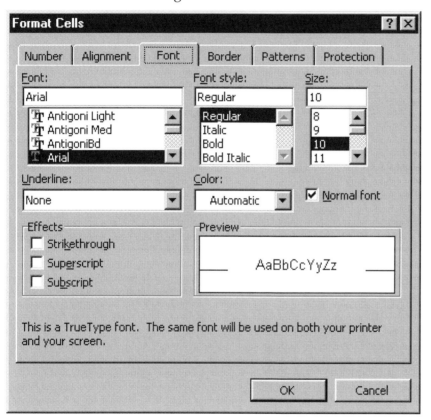

Exercise

As an exercise, see if you can restore the entire table to Arial 10pt Bold using the dialog box.

Formatting numbers

There are many formatting features for dealing with numbers in Excel. Rather than deal with them all here, we will simply point out that as usual they can be accessed via the toolbar or the menus, and then deal with a few of the more important points relevant to this scenario.

The formatting toolbar has five buttons relevant to numbers:

which in turn, from left to right relate to:

• currency format

• percentage format

• commas between thousands

• increase decimal places by one

• decrease decimal places by one.

In our scenario, we use some of these to help us provide more detail on our attendances. First, we are going to add a further column to our table:

🖰 **Click** on E3

⌨️ **Type** =D3/C3↵

to calculate the over or under utilisation as a fraction of the planned provision.

🖰 **Click** on E3.

🖰 **AutoFill** down from E3 to E14.

With the cells still highlighted:

🖰 **Click** on %.

The fraction is converted to a percentage.

To add one decimal place:

🖰 **Click** on ⚏ ..

To add another:

🖰 **Click** on ⚏ again.

To reduce it back to one:

🖰 **Click** on ⚏.

We will deal with the others when we come to financial matters.

To access the functions available via the menu:

🖰 **Click** on Format in the menu bar

🖰 **Click** on Cells in the Format menu

🖰 **Click** on the Number tab.

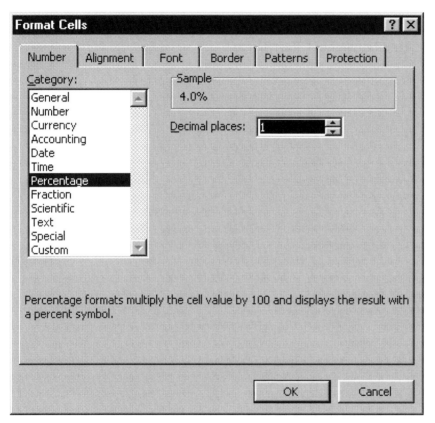

As we have nothing to add at this point:

🖰 **Click** on Cancel to close the dialog box.

We will meet the other formats in other scenarios.

One of the quirky things about Excel (well I think it's quirky, but there are people who say I'm quirky myself) is how to remove those gridlines that shout 'I'M A SPREADSHEET'.

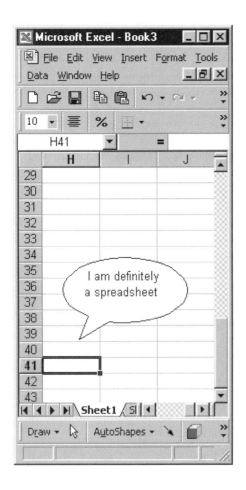

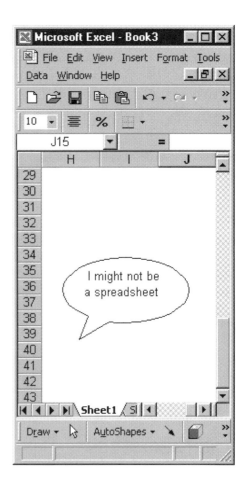

Hint

The gridlines are not printed, the following only applies to the screen display.

It's quirky because it's located on the Tools menu.

🖱 **Click** on Tools in the menu bar

🖱 **Click** on Options.

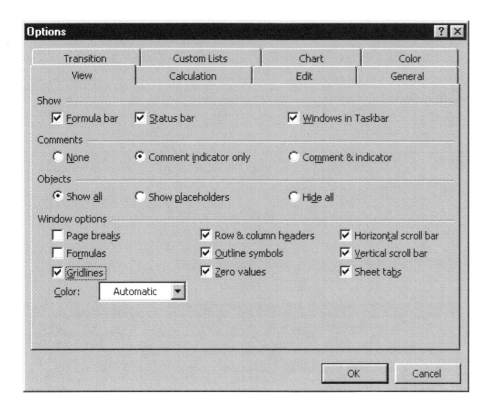

The dialog box gives access to a vast range of customisation options:

 Click on the View tab

 Click on Gridlines

 Click on ⬚ OK ⬚ .

Hint

The View gridlines option is an example of a toggle option, i.e. it's either on or off. You have encountered these before, with things like the Bold and Italic toolbar buttons. However, this option is explicitly shown as ☑ (on) or ☐ (off). As with text formatting, clicking in the box reverses the switch.

Borders

Having removed the gridlines, we may still want to highlight certain areas by use of a border:

🖰 **Highlight** the area A1 to F15 (to ensure the title fits within the border)

🖰 **Click** on ⊞ ▾ in the tool bar.

This produces a range of border options:

🖰 **Click** on the bottom right-hand option.

A simple border will now surround the highlighted area. The result is shown below. The border button changes as the border itself changes.

Once again, for complete flexibility, we can use the menu by selecting the Border tab from the F<u>o</u>rmat C<u>e</u>lls dialog box, accessed from the F<u>o</u>rmat menu.

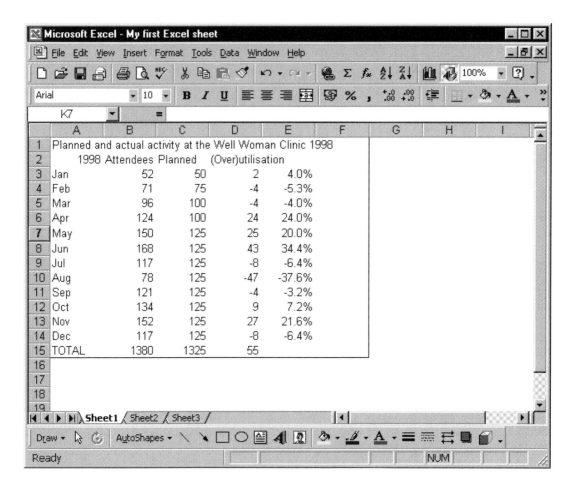

Well that just about concludes the sums bit. There are just a few bits you might like to try.

If we want to print the sheet, the easiest way is to use the print button on the toolbar:

🖱 **Click** on 🖨 .

However, it is generally worth having a look at the result first on the screen. To achieve this:

🖱 **Click** on 🔍 (print preview) which is next to the Print button on the toolbar.

This allows us to preview what the printed version will look like. Note that the pointer changes to a magnifying glass:

🖱 **Click** on Setup … and we can change almost anything about the way the sheet is printed.

The available options are accessed by a dialog box with four tabs:

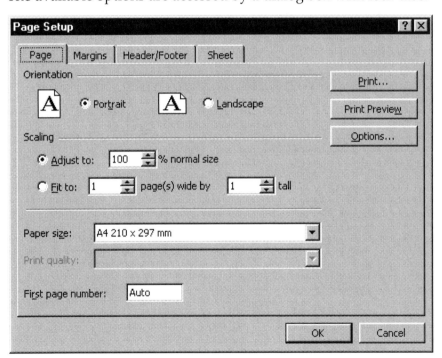

One of the most useful options is the scaling option which allows us either to specify a scaling factor or to fit the sheet automatically to a number of pages. Note that all changes are shown on the preview screen.

Exercise

As the printing options are not safety critical, they are left for the reader to explore as an exercise. Use it to see how confident you are moving around in Excel.

To leave Setup either

🖱 **Click** on ⬚ OK ⬚ to save the options as set, or

🖱 **Click** on ⬚ Cancel ⬚ to close the dialog box without saving the options set.

Once the Setup options are set, then the worksheet may be printed from within the main preview dialog box:

🖱 **Click** on Print.

The Print dialog box appears:

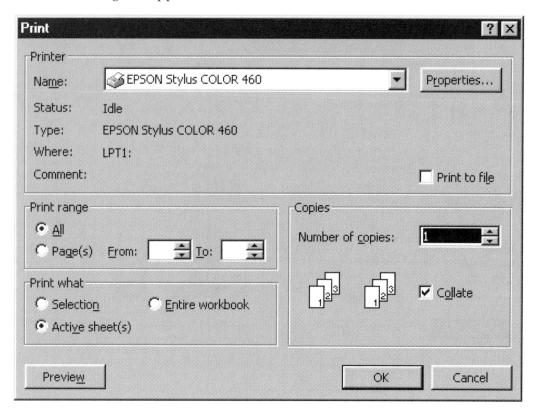

Health warning

The name of the printer in use will appear at the top of the box next to the word printer, e.g. Epson Stylus Color 460 in my case.

Fortunately, most printing goes very smoothly and problems arise when ink or paper runs out – **CHECK THIS FIRST**! If this doesn't work, then remember that printing in Excel is controlled by Windows, not Excel. However, if you experience problems the first port of call is the Properties button, and the screen behind it, shown below.

After this you will need to go back to your Windows set-up. Time to reach for your yellow book!

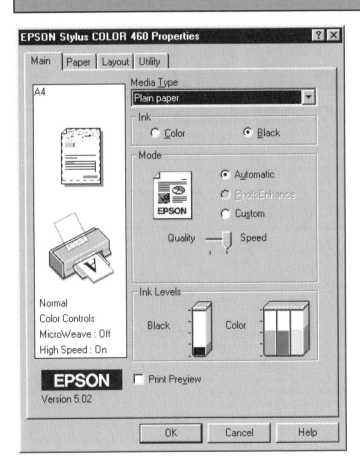

Back at the Print dialog box itself, we have options to print a selection, a sheet or the entire collection of sheets known as a workbook. Within this, we have the option to print all the pages or a selected range. The buttons on the right allow us to access the preview facility, or to change the page or printer set-up.

If the printer is set up correctly and the page is set up according to our wishes, then all we need to do is:

🖱 **Click** on ⬜ OK ⬜ to print our sheet.

You should now save your sheet. But of course you've been doing that all the way through, haven't you?

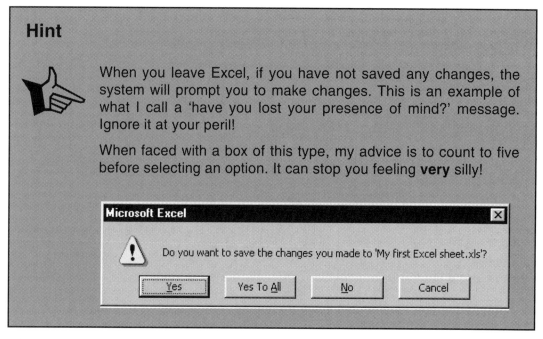

Hint

When you leave Excel, if you have not saved any changes, the system will prompt you to make changes. This is an example of what I call a 'have you lost your presence of mind?' message. Ignore it at your peril!

When faced with a box of this type, my advice is to count to five before selecting an option. It can stop you feeling **very** silly!

Now suppose you want to illustrate your work to colleagues in the practice. Wouldn't it be nice to have a pretty graph to show them?

I think that the graphs are one of the neatest bits of Excel. The temptation however is to over-egg them. It really doesn't matter whether that bar is magenta or purple. Well, I would say that – I'm colour blind!

The first graph we consider is one of the number of attendees:

🖱 **Highlight** A2 to B14

🖱 **Click** on 📊 to invoke the Chart Wizard.

The Chart Wizard is a four-step process to plot a wide range of graphs. We start by trying to draw a simple two-dimensional column chart.

Hint

 Excel calls what most of us call a bar chart, a column chart. In Excel, if the bars are vertical, it's a column chart; if they're horizontal, it's a bar chart. There is a sort of logic!

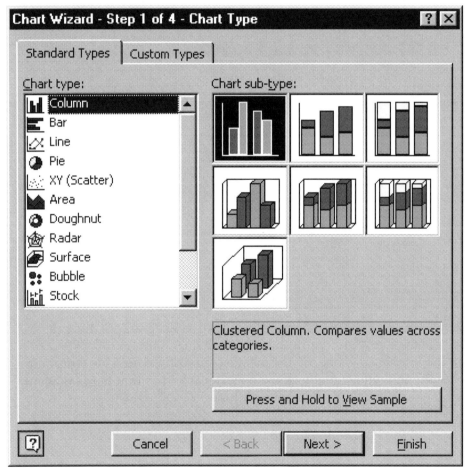

🖰 **Click** on Next >.

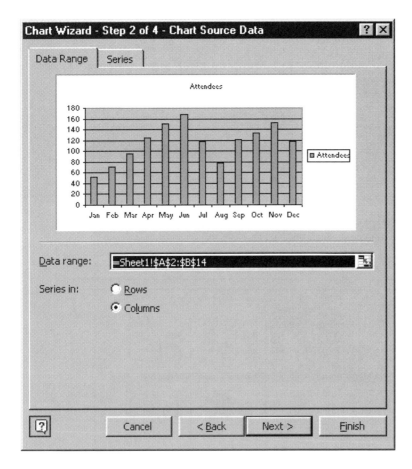

☝ **Click** on Next >.

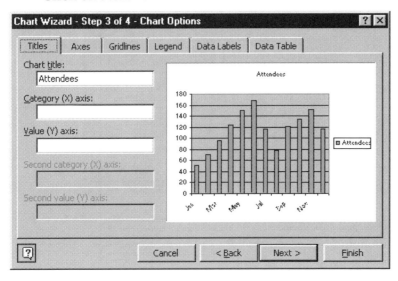

🖱 **Click** on Next >.

🖱 **Click** on As new sheet.

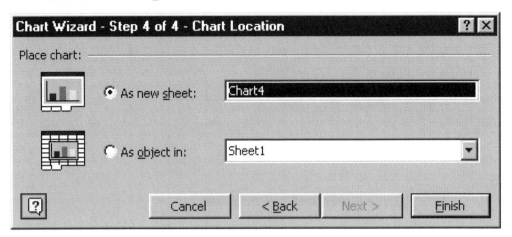

🖱 **Click** on Finish.

The chart is now complete. The result is shown below:

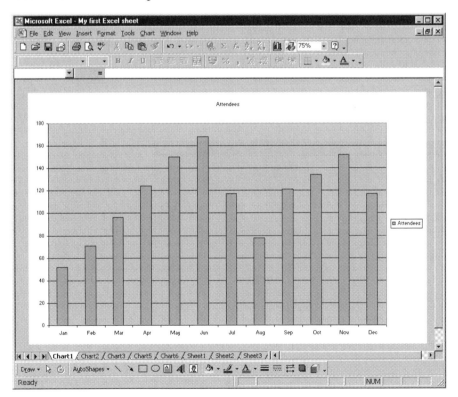

Health warning

Excel often produces a chart that is very pretty, but not strictly accurate. For example, here the column chart implies that there is a gap between each month. In practice, as each month is continuous from the last one, there should be no gaps between the columns.

We now produce another graph of the same data, being a bit more selective. Specifically, we choose options to:

- produce a 3-D column chart
- put attendees as the Y-Axis title
- add the contents of A1 as the main title
- select a transparent background
- delete the legend
- make the gridlines dashed
- align the text on the vertical axis vertically.

OK, so here goes:

🖱 **Click** on the Sheet1 tab

🖱 **Highlight** A1 to B14

🖱 **Click** on 📊 to invoke the Chart Wizard.

🖱 **Click** on 📊

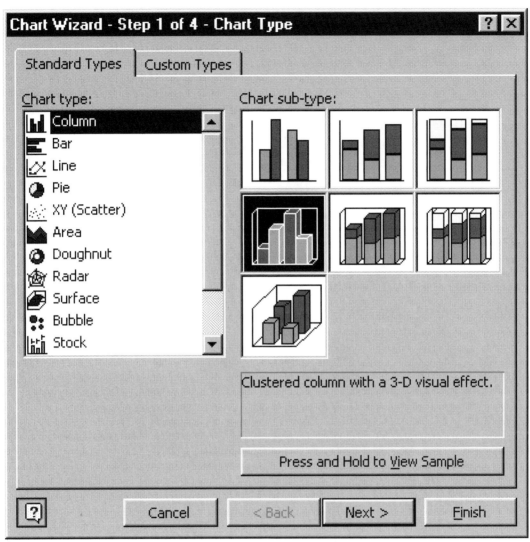

🖰 **Click** on Next >

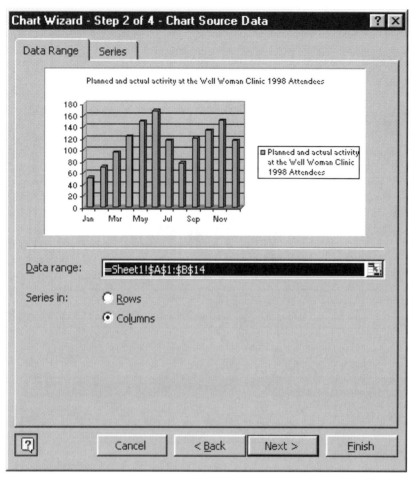

🖑 **Click** on Next >

🖑 **Click** in the Chart title box to produce a flashing cursor

⌨ **Press** [End] to go to the end

🖑 **Highlight** Attendees

⌨ **Hold** [Ctrl] and **Press** X to cut Attendees

⌨ **Press** [tab] twice to get to the Value (Z) Axis box

⌨ **Hold** [Ctrl] and **Press** V to paste Attendees here

🖑 **Click** on the Legend tab

🖑 **Click** in the Show Legend box to remove the legend

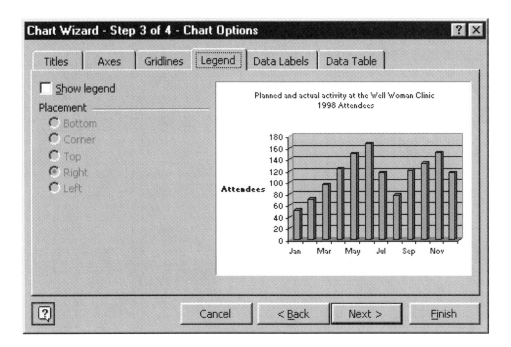

🖰 **Click** on Next >

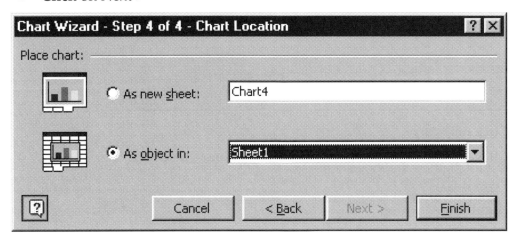

🖰 **Click** on As new sheet

🖰 **Click** on Finish.

The chart is now complete and the result is shown below:

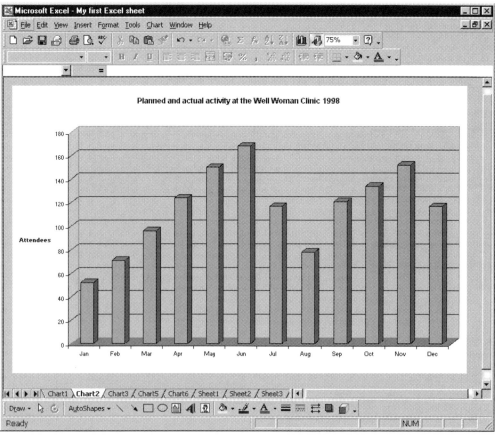

We can still tidy up a few details.

To remove the grey background:

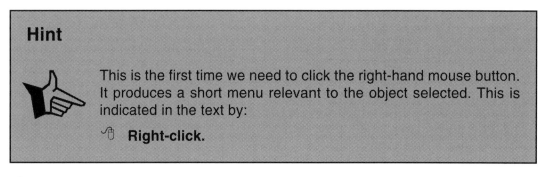

🖰 **Right-click** on the background

Hint

This is the first time we need to click the right-hand mouse button. It produces a short menu relevant to the object selected. This is indicated in the text by:

🖰 **Right-click.**

🖰 **Click** on Format Walls

🖰 **Click** on None in the Area box

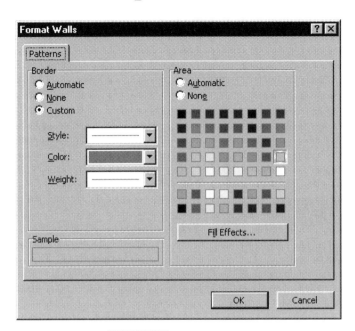

🖰 **Click** on [OK].

To make the gridlines dashed:

🖰 **Right-click** on a gridline

🖰 **Click** on Format Gridlines

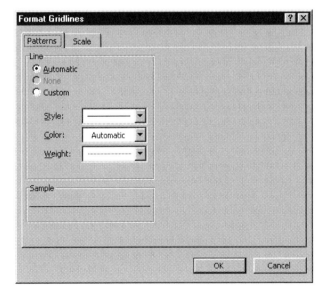

🖰 **Click** on ▾ in the Style list.

From the resulting list:

🖰 **Click** on the dashed style

🖰 **Click** on ▭ OK ▭ .

Finally, to align the text vertically on the vertical axis:

🖰 **Right-click** on the axis label.

🖰 **Click** on Format Axis Title

🖰 **Click** on the Alignment tab

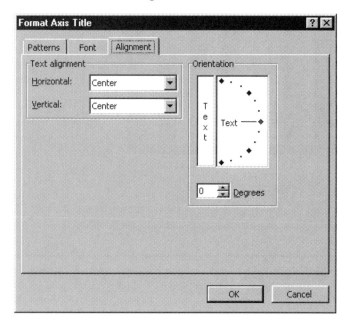

🖰 **Click** in the Degrees number box before the zero

⌨ **Type** a 9 to change the angle to 90°.

🖰 **Click** on ▭ OK ▭ .

The result is shown below:

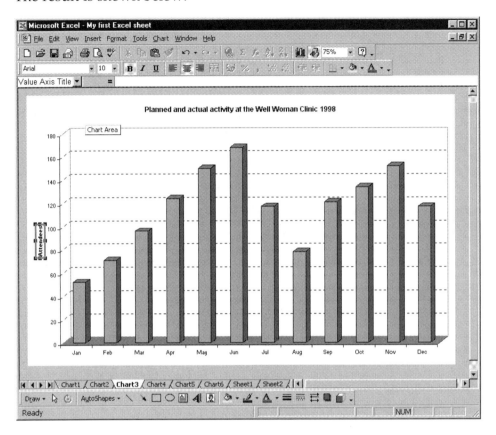

Exercise

There are three more graphs to plot within this scenario:

1 Graph of over-utilisation by month in absolute terms.
2 Graph of over-utilisation by month in percentage terms.
3 Graph comparing planned and actual utilisation.

These are left as an exercise for the reader with some broad hints overleaf.

Hint

You need to remember how to highlight two separate sections of a sheet. If you didn't read the section *Before we start*, now is the time!

For example, for graph 1 you need to highlight A2 to A14 and D2 to D14 before invoking the Chart Wizard.

The trick is to use the [Ctrl] key!

There now follow three model answers as to how the graphs might look. Each model answer shows the areas highlighted to produce the resulting charts. All you have to do is to get from one to the other!

	A	B	C	D	E	F	G
1	Planned and actual activity at the Well Woman Clinic 1998						
2	1998	Attendees	Planned	(Over)utilisation			
3	Jan	52	50	2	4.0%		
4	Feb	71	75	-4	-5.3%		
5	Mar	96	100	-4	-4.0%		
6	Apr	124	100	24	24.0%		
7	May	150	125	25	20.0%		
8	Jun	168	125	43	34.4%		
9	Jul	117	125	-8	-6.4%		
10	Aug	78	125	-47	-37.6%		
11	Sep	121	125	-4	-3.2%		
12	Oct	134	125	9	7.2%		
13	Nov	152	125	27	21.6%		
14	Dec	117	125	-8	-6.4%		
15	TOTAL	1380	1325	55			
16							

Chart2 / Chart3 / Chart4 / Chart5 / Ch

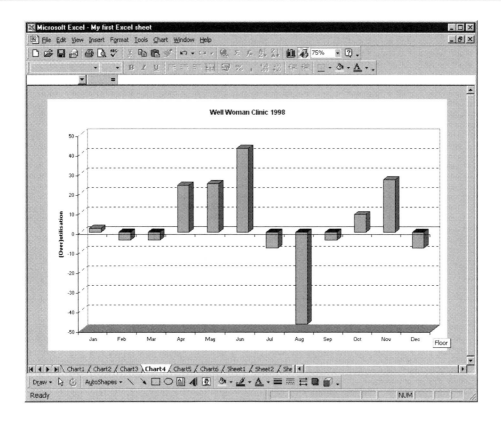

	A	B	C	D	E	F	G
1	Planned and actual activity at the Well Woman Clinic 1998						
2	1998	Attendees	Planned	(Over)utilisation			
3	Jan	52	50	2	4.0%		
4	Feb	71	75	-4	-5.3%		
5	Mar	96	100	-4	-4.0%		
6	Apr	124	100	24	24.0%		
7	May	150	125	25	20.0%		
8	Jun	168	125	43	34.4%		
9	Jul	117	125	-8	-6.4%		
10	Aug	78	125	-47	-37.6%		
11	Sep	121	125	-4	-3.2%		
12	Oct	134	125	9	7.2%		
13	Nov	152	125	27	21.6%		
14	Dec	117	125	-8	-6.4%		
15	TOTAL	1380	1325	55			
16							

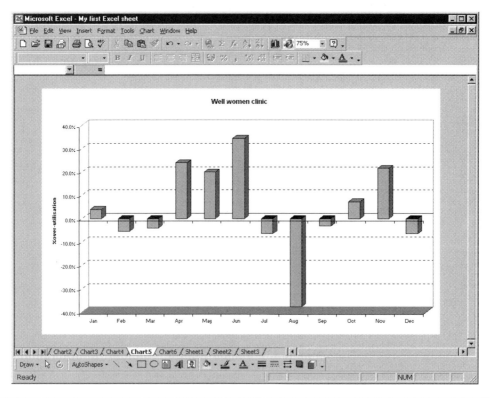

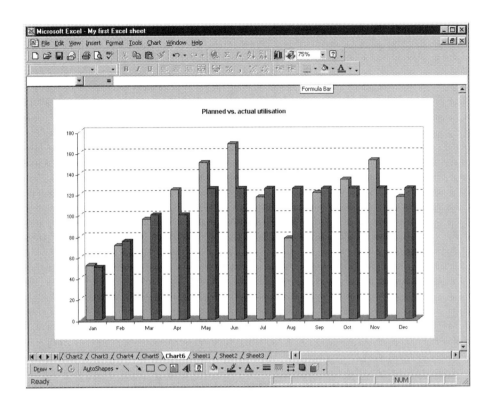

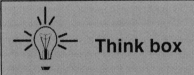 **Think box**

Once you have drawn the graphs consider the following questions:

1 What does each graph actually convey?

2 Which graph communicates the best?

3 What are the implications for future service within the clinic?

Governance scenario 2

Child health monitoring in primary and community care

In this chapter

This chapter will tell you how to:

- monitor levels of attendance at developmental checks
- monitor the uptake of immunisations
- produce a quantitative performance measure

 use Excel as a simple database

 process data as dates and fractions

 sort and search data

 use logical formulae

 introduce comments associated with cells.

The scenario

A practice of four partners (one half time) with a total list size of 6430 patients is concerned to ensure that children within their practice in the first year of life are receiving the best possible care.

They have set up a monitoring system to evaluate practice performance in terms of ensuring that the target children attend for their immunisations and regular check-ups.

The aim is to produce performance indicators in key areas to monitor performance.

Child monitoring system

We start by showing how Excel can be used as a simple way of looking at patient records.

Excel is no substitute for a sophisticated database package but it provides some database handling functions that can be useful.

To start:

🖱 **Open** Child health monitoring.

Hint

From now on in the text we use the instruction 'Open' to refer to the task of opening a new sheet. This is equivalent to:

🖱 **Click** on File on the menu bar

🖱 **Click** on Open

🖱 **Select** Child health monitoring

🖱 **Click** on [OK]

or in its briefest form

🖱 **Click** on 🗁

🖱 **Double-click** on Child health monitoring.

The Open dialog box looks something like the one below:

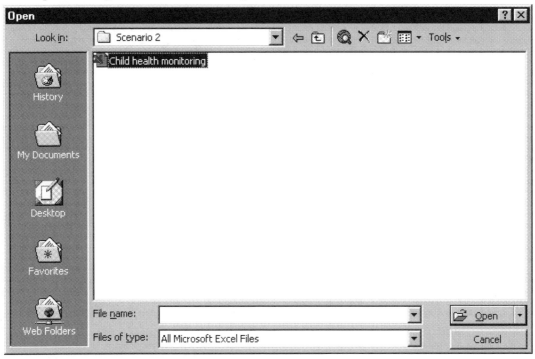

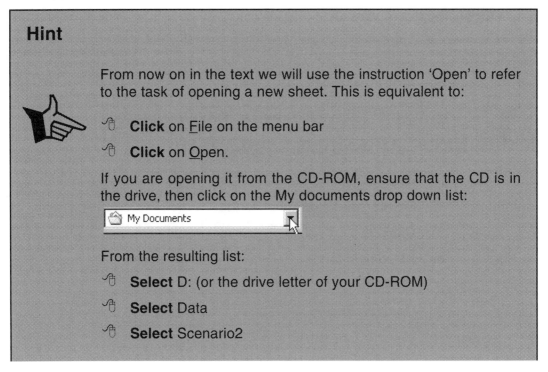

Hint

From now on in the text we will use the instruction 'Open' to refer to the task of opening a new sheet. This is equivalent to:

- **Click** on File on the menu bar
- **Click** on Open.

If you are opening it from the CD-ROM, ensure that the CD is in the drive, then click on the My documents drop down list:

From the resulting list:

- **Select** D: (or the drive letter of your CD-ROM)
- **Select** Data
- **Select** Scenario2

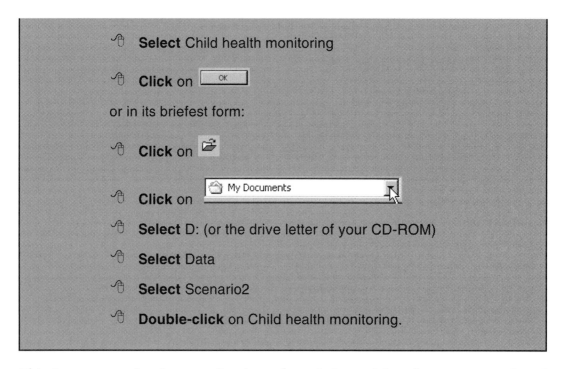

This is an example of an application where it is useful to have numerical and graphical functions available in a data handling application. The system holds data on the target population of 98 infants concerning their birth and inoculation histories. It will be used to monitor performance in this area and produce performance indicators. To find out how the data may be transferred from your practice system, look to the Appendix at the end of this book.

Using Excel as a simple database

Excel makes use of the concept of data lists. A list is a column with a title in the first row and data in each of the other rows. Excel treats the first row as a header and allows you to identify the column by the text in the first row. It also ignores the first row when sorting data or carrying out similar operations. This makes the use of Excel as a simple database simpler than some other spreadsheets, including early versions of Excel.

Health warning

Excel will automatically treat data as lists, providing that at least one cell is selected within the region where the dataset is stored. Always click on a cell before using data functions to ensure that they work correctly.

The first row of the sheet contains a list of headers describing the data contained in each column.

The lists in the child monitoring system.

Column	Header	Data stored
A	Surname:	contains the patients' surnames
B	Forenames:	contains the patients' forenames
C	Sex:	contains the patients' sex
D	DOB:	contains the patients' dates of birth
E	Birth weight:	contains the patients' weight, stored as a fraction
F	6-week check:	contains the date that the patients attended for their 6-week check; blank indicates non-attendance
G	Triple 1:	contains the date that the patients attended for their first triple immunisation; blank indicates non-attendance
H	Triple 2:	contains the date that the patients attended for their second triple immunisation; blank indicates non-attendance
I	Triple 3:	contains the date that the patients attended for their third triple immunisation; blank indicates non-attendance
J	7-month check:	contains the date that the patients attended for their 7-month check; blank indicates non-attendance
K	12-month MMR:	contains the date that the patients attended for their MMR (Mumps, Measles and Rubella) injection at 12 months; blank indicates non-attendance

Before we use the system in anger, we will copy the data into a new worksheet in the same workbook. This is good practice, as it ensures that the original dataset is left intact.

 Principle of good practice

Always leave a safe copy of your original data, and work on a copy. This will ensure that the original is intact. This may be achieved by copying the data to a separate sheet in the same workbook.

This is no substitute for proper back-ups which should be taken anyway!

To take a copy of the data:

🖲 **Highlight** cells A1 to K97

🖲 **Click** on 📑 in the toolbar to copy the selected cells

🖲 **Click** on the tab at the bottom marked 'Sheet3' to select a new sheet

🖲 **Click** on cell A1

🖲 **Click on** 📋 in the toolbar to paste the selected cells into the new sheet.

Don't worry if you get lots of #####s. This simply means that the columns aren't wide enough. To fix this:

🖲 **Click** on Format to select the format menu

🖲 **Click** on Column to select the column sub-menu

🖲 **Click** on AutoFit Selection to fit the columns better.

Now we have a copy of our data to work on.

One feature of this system is that there are many different types of data. For example, Columns D and G to K contain data in date format. To see how this is done, we format a blank column in the same way:

🖲 **Click** on the header to column L to highlight the whole column

🖲 **Click** on Format from the menu bar

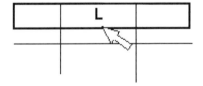

🖱 **Click** on Cells

🖱 **Click** on the Number tab (if not already selected)

🖱 **Click** on Date in the list of categories

🖱 **Click** on 'dd-mmm-yy' in the list of Format Codes

🖱 **Click** on [OK] .

Birth weight presents a problem as it is generally recorded in pounds and ounces. This can be handled by using the fraction format. In the sheet provided, Column E is formatted as a fraction. If the data points are input as decimals, then it is displayed as fractions allowing the ounces to appear as sixteenths of pounds.

To see how this was done, re-format Column L as follows:

🖱 **Click** on Format to select format menu

🖱 **Click** on Cells

🖱 **Click** on the Number tab (if not already selected)

🖱 **Click** on Fraction in the list of categories

🖱 **Click** on As sixteenths (8/16) in the list of categories

🖱 **Click** on [OK] .

Excel allows us to look at individual records as well as the overall table view. To look at an individual patient record:

🖱 **Click** on A2 (this can be any cell with data in it)

🖱 **Click** on Data from the menu bar

🖱 **Click** on Form.

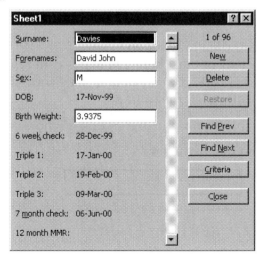

Health warning

The actual dates displayed will differ from those shown here. Do not panic! This is a side effect of providing an exercise that continually updates itself.

The data displayed as record 1 is stored in row 2 of our sheet, because row 1 contains the header information.

We can use the Find facility to find a specific patient record:

🖱 **Click** on Criteria

⌨ **Type** Gillies in the ⎵⎵⎵⎵⎵ next to Surname

🖱 **Click** on ⎡ Find Next ⎤ .

This takes us to our required record.

We can also use the form to add new records:

🖱 **Click** on ⎡ New ⎤ .

This brings up a blank record:

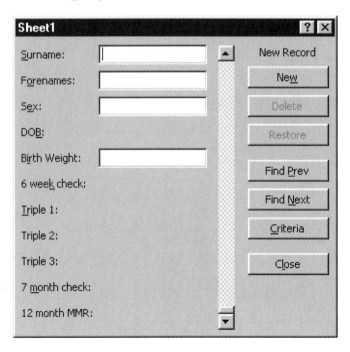

This cannot be filled in. We will use it for practice:

 Type Green in the <u>S</u>urname box

Hint

 The tab key is a really convenient way to move between fields. However, see the health warning below.

 Press [tab] to move to the next field.

☢ Health warning

Pressing ⏎ before the completion of data entry will cause data entry to cease!

At the completion of each box use a [tab] key **not** a ⏎ (enter) key to move to the next field. At the completion of the whole form, use a ⏎ key to complete the data entry for that record.

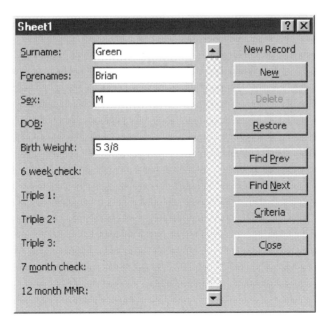

Fill in the rest of the fields as shown below, using the tab key to move between fields, and substituting today's actual date for the DO<u>B</u> field.

Once these fields are complete:

🖱 **Click** on C<u>l</u>ose.

The new record appears in row 98 of our sheet.

In order to preserve the integrity of our original data, we will delete this record. First, we get our form back:

🖱 **Click** on <u>D</u>ata from the menu bar

🖱 **Click** on F<u>o</u>rm.

Next we need to find the record:

🖱 **Click** on <u>C</u>riteria

⌨ **Type** Green in the [   ] next to Surname

🖱 **Click** on Find Next.

This takes us to the next instance of a patient with the surname Green. However, this is not the required record:

🖱 **Click** on Find Next again, and until Record 97 of 97 is reached.

🖱 **Click** on Delete to delete the record.

Sorting data

The List facility where Excel identifies each column by the label in the first row allows us to use the sort function to sort data into ascending or descending order. The sort procedure is based on the use of one or more columns as the 'key' field, identified by the label in row 1. In this particular example, we will use the Date of Birth as the key by which the records will be sorted:

🖱 **Click** on any cell in Column D

🖱 **Click** on <u>D</u>ata from the menu bar

🖱 **Click** on <u>S</u>ort.

Because we selected a cell in Column D, Excel assumes that we would like to sort the data by Date of Birth.

The dialog box that appears should look like the one below:

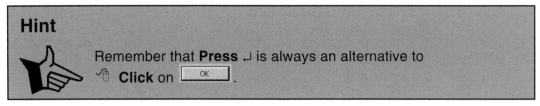

To sort, simply:

⌐🖰 **Click** on ⟨ OK ⟩.

> # Hint
>
> Remember that **Press** ⏎ is always an alternative to
> ⌐🖰 **Click** on ⟨ OK ⟩.

The records are now sorted by date of birth.

Now we try a more sophisticated sort where the records are sorted by Sex, Surname and Forename in that order. The records are required to be listed with boys first, then in alphabetical order of surname and then forenames. This involves the use of three keys, the order in which the columns are put in the key dialog box determining the sort order:

⌐🖰 **Click** on any cell in Column A

⌐🖰 **Click** on Data from the menu bar

⌐🖰 **Click** on Sort.

This puts up the Sort dialog box with Sex filled in as the first field to sort on. To put the boys first (Why? Because it's a nasty sexist world – actually because it illustrates a teaching point, honestly!):

⌐🖰 **Click** on Descending (M comes after F)

⌐🖰 **Click** on ▼ in the first Then by box

⌐🖰 **Click** on Surname in the resulting list

⌐🖰 **Click** on Forenames in the resulting list.

The sort box should look like:

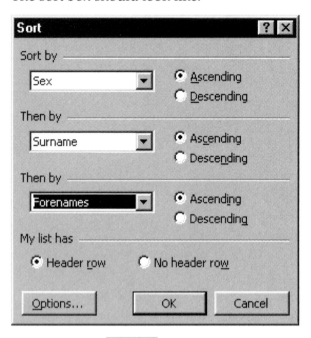

Click on [OK] to sort the records into boys, then girls. Amongst each gender group, the records are sorted into alphabetical order of surname. Where this is common, the Christian names are used to order the records.

The effect can be seen by looking at the cells in the range A46 to C63 which illustrate all of these effects:

	A	B	C
46	Smith	Duncan John	M
47	Smith	Stephen James	M
48	Steel	Stephen Christopher	M
49	Taylor	Stephen John	M
50	Tomlinson	Mark	M
51	Turner	James Alexander	M
52	Wainwright	Paul Eliot	M
53	Watkinson	Stephen Michael	M
54	Watts	Clive David	M
55	Webster	Paul David	M
56	Wesley	Colin Stephen	M
57	West	Peter Graham	M
58	Wilcock	Gordon James	M
59	Wilson	Simon John	M
60	Abbott	Emma Jane	F
61	Armfield	Naomi Catherine	F
62	Armstrong	Sara Ann	F
63	Atkinson	Sally Christine	F

Filtering data

As well as sorting data, Excel provides the facility to filter out a specific group of records. Supposing, for example, we want to select only the female children:

🖱 **Click** on cell C2

🖱 **Click** on <u>D</u>ata from the menu bar

🖱 **Click** on <u>F</u>ilter

🖱 **Click** on Auto<u>F</u>ilter.

In the first row of each column, a ▾ appears to signify a drop down menu:

🖱 **Click** on ▾ next to Sex in cell C1

🖱 **Click** on F in the resulting list.

Only the data relating to the female patients is shown. To view only a particular patient, select their surname:

🖱 **Click** on ▾ next to Surname in cell A1

🖱 **Click** on Gillies in the resulting list.

If the surname does not uniquely identify a record, then we can use combinations of filters. For example, to select John Smith, first restore all the data:

🖱 **Click** on ▾ next to Surname in cell A1

🖱 **Click** on (All) in the resulting list

🖱 **Click** on ▾ next to Sex in cell C1

🖱 **Click** on (All) in the resulting list.

Now to select John Smith:

🖱 **Click** on ▾ next to Surname in cell A1

🖱 **Click** on Smith in the resulting list

🖱 **Click** on ▾ next to Sex in cell C1

🖱 **Click** on John Frederick in the resulting list.

Suppose we want to find the non-attenders for the first triple injection. We can use the (blanks) option.

First restore all the data:

🖱 **Click** on ▾ next to Surname in cell A1

🖱 **Click** on (All) in the resulting list

🖱 **Click** on ⬛ next to Forename in cell B1.

Now to identify the non-attenders:

🖱 **Click** on ⬛ next to Triple1 in cell G1

🖱 **Click** on (blanks) at the bottom of the resulting list.

This tells us that three children have not attended for this injection. However, some of these children may be too young to attend yet. To filter a set of data and specify a range of values, we use the custom criteria option. For example, to find all those children weighing over 7lbs at birth, first restore all the data:

🖱 **Click** on ⬛ next to Triple1 in cell G1

🖱 **Click** on (All) in the resulting list.

Now to identify the heavier babies:

🖱 **Click** on ⬛ next to Birth Weight in cell E1

🖱 **Click** on (Custom) in the resulting list.

This produces the following dialog box:

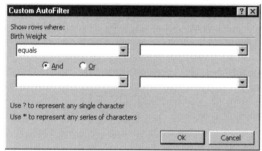

🖱 **Click** on ⬛ next to equals.

🖱 **Click** on greater than in the resulting list

⌨ **Press** →|

⌨ **Type** 7 (this corresponds to a birth weight of 7lbs)

🖱 **Click** on ⬛ OK ⬛.

Excel now displays those babies with birth weights greater than 7lbs.
    To leave AutoFilter mode:

🖱 **Click** on Data from the menu bar

🖱 **Click** on Filter

🖰 **Click** on Auto<u>F</u>ilter.

The AutoFilter facility is switched off and the drop down menu arrows disappear.

Searching for and replacing data

The way to find specific data (without using a form) is to use the search and replace facility, which works in a similar way to search and replace on a word processor. To find a cell containing a specific piece of data, say 'Ivor', we can use the Find facility. Notice that the value to be found does not have to be the whole cell value:

🖰 **Click** on <u>E</u>dit from the menu bar

🖰 **Click** on <u>F</u>ind

⌨ **Type** Ivor↲.

The Find dialog box is shown below.

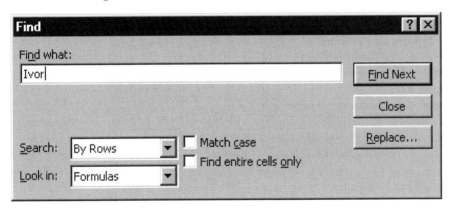

🖰 **Click** on ⬚ Close ⬚.

The cell containing the search text is highlighted.

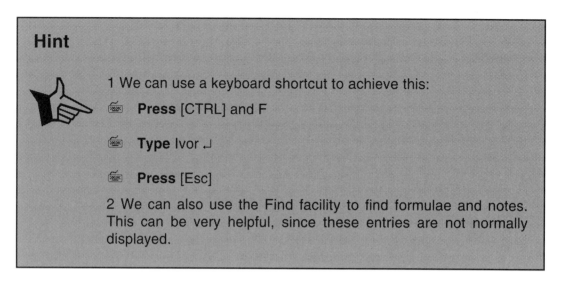

Hint

1 We can use a keyboard shortcut to achieve this:

⌨ **Press** [CTRL] and F

⌨ **Type** Ivor ↵

⌨ **Press** [Esc]

2 We can also use the Find facility to find formulae and notes. This can be very helpful, since these entries are not normally displayed.

It is also possible to search for and replace data in a particular cell:

🖰 **Click** on Edit from the menu bar

🖰 **Click** on Replace.

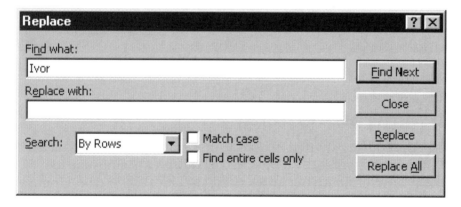

⌨ **Type** M↵.

Note that typing replaces the highlighted 'Ivor'.

🖰 Click in the ☐ below 'Replace with'.

At the flashing cursor in the box:

⌨ **Type** Male

🖰 **Click** on ☑ next to 'Find entire cells only'.

Health warning

If you miss out this stage, you will find strange values appearing like 'Maleonth'!

🖱 **Click** on [Find Next] .

🖱 **Click** on [Replace All] .

Now try to repeat the process yourself, to substitute Female for F.

Hint

You may need to change the column width to accommodate 'Female': refer back to earlier in the chapter if you can't remember how to do it.

Performance measurement

Excel is very good at producing quantitative measures from qualitative data and displaying these measures graphically. Thus, Excel can be a significant tool in producing quantitative performance measures within a clinical governance framework.

First, we consider some simple quantitative functions.

The average function

We can provide information on the average (mean) birth weight of the children with the following:

🖱 **Click** on D98

⌨ **Type** Mean

Click on E98.

 Click on *f* on the toolbar (this is the Function Wizard).

Hint

Functions are very important in Excel. They consist of two bits. The *function* itself defines *what it does*, e.g. average, sum, sin, today, etc. The *parameters* define *what it does it to*, usually a cell or range of cells, in this case E2 to E98.

The Function Wizard consists of two dialog boxes, one to select the function, the next to select the parameters, as illustrated below.

If we are lucky, the function is one used recently, in which case it appears in the list on the right-hand side in the Most Recently Used category. The average is a commonly used function and should be there.

If so:

 Click on Average in the list.

Otherwise:

 Click on Statistical in the list of function categories and then

 Click on Average in the list.

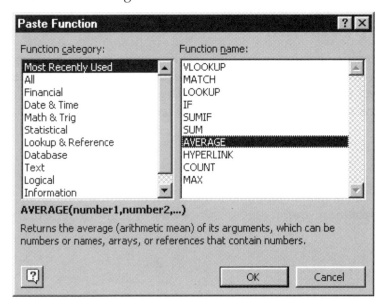

🖰 **Click** on ⬚ ᴏᴋ ⬚ .

At this point, Excel gets clever and decides that you want the average of the data above the formula. So it fills in the range of cells to be averaged all by itself (scary, huh?). In fairness, it does give you the chance to change it.

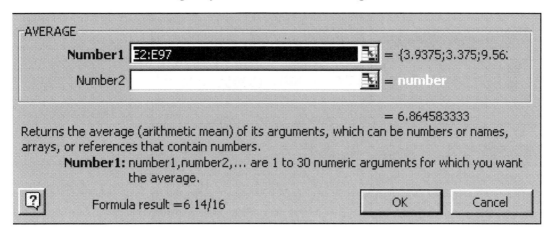

🖰 **Click** on ⬚ ᴏᴋ ⬚ to accept Excel's judgement.

Just to prove that it really is a smart alec, it even quotes the answer in sixteenths to match the data. The correct answer is 6lbs 14oz for the data as given. At least the computer doesn't know what ounces are!

The standard deviation

We can go one step further in sophistication by providing some information on the dispersion of the birth weights around the average or mean value. In a large sample, we would expect 68% of the birth weights to be within plus or minus one standard deviation of the mean, and 95% to be within two standard deviations.

🖰 **Click** on D99.

⌨ **Type** St.Dev.

🖰 **Click** on E19.

🖰 **Click** on *fₓ* in the toolbar.

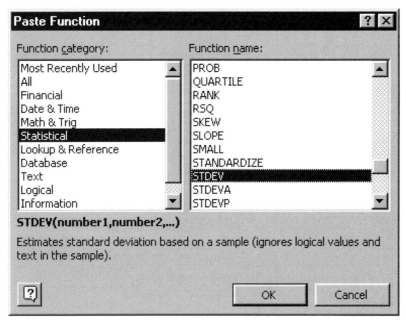

Once again, if we are lucky, the function is one used recently, in which case it appears in the list on the right-hand side in the Most Recently Used category.

The standard deviation is less likely to be there than the average:

🖱 **Click** on Statistical in the list of function categories and then

🖱 **Click** on the list of statistical functions

⌨ **Press** S to go down to functions beginning with S.

Scroll down to the standard deviation functions:

🖱 **Click** on STDEV in the list.

🖱 **Click** on ⬛ OK ⬛.

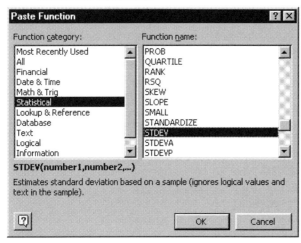

Once again, Excel tries to guess the range. Only this time it gets it wrong! Excel 1 User 1.

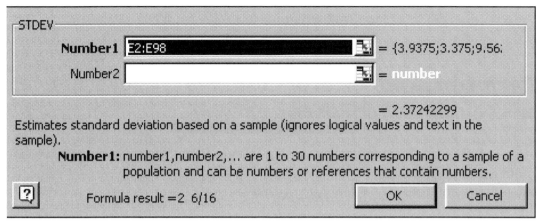

To adjust the formula to its correct value E2:E97, not E2:E98, we:

🖰 **Click** to the right of the 8.

At the flashing cursor:

⌨ **Press** ← (Backspace key)

⌨ **Press** 7.

The formula should now read E2:E97.

🖰 Click on [OK].

Health warning

There are four functions for the standard deviation in Excel: STDEV and STDEVP giving the sample and population standard deviations respectively, and each comes in standard (STDEV/STDEVP) and deluxe versions (STDEVA/STDEVPA).

It is essential that you use the correct version. Where your dataset is small and a sample of the total population is clearly under investigation, then use the sample standard deviation (STDEV). The difference between sample and population versions decreases as the sample size increases, i.e. as the sample approaches the total population.

The deluxe versions (STDEVA/STDEVPA) are Excel variants to take account of text and logical values – an irrelevance in most cases.

Rule 1: If in doubt consult a passing statistician.

Rule 2: If there isn't one passing at the time, go and find one!

The correct answer is 2.38 for the data as given. The computer will quote a ludicrous number of decimal places. To reduce them to a precision comparable to your data, and justified by the technique used, click on the decrease decimal toolbar button (   )with cell E98 selected until only two decimal places are showing.

Performance indicators for clinical governance: percentage of children reached

We would like to keep track of how many children are being immunised and to see what percentage of the children we are reaching. This can be done, but it is not quite as simple as it might appear. First, we need to work out how many children are being immunised or are attending clinics:

🖰 **Click** on B98

⌨ **Type** Total recorded

🖰 **Click** on C98

🖰 **Click** on *fx* in the toolbar.

If not already selected:

🖰 **Click** on Statistical in the list of function categories

🖰 **Click** on ▼ a few times beside the statistical functions to scroll down to COUNTA

🖰 **Click** on COUNTA in the list of statistical functions (it's just below the bottom of the first page of functions)

🖰 **Click** on ☐ OK ☐.

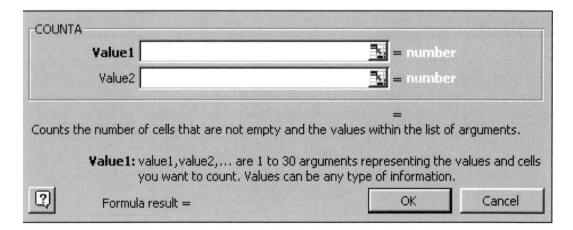

This time, perhaps discouraged by previous failures, Excel doesn't even try to enter a range.

⌨ **Type** C2:C97.

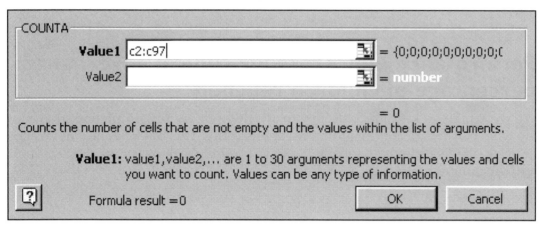

⌨ **Press** ↵.

Excel counts the number of entries in this column, corresponding to the number of children (96).

Now we use the same formula to calculate the number of attendances for check-ups or immunisations:

🖱 **AutoFill** the formula across from C98 to K98.

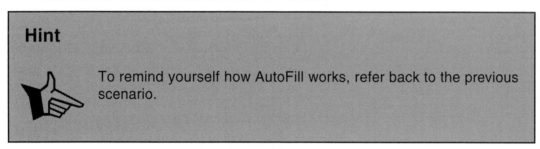

This gives us our first measure of performance: the number of children attending for a check-up or immunisation. However, performance is judged as a percentage of the total target population. This total varies according to how old the children are on any specific day.

Hint

It's that word 'population' again. Here we are using it in the sense of the group of patients identified as the target by our screening protocol.

For Columns C to E, the answer is the total population, and therefore we can easily set these:

🖱 **Click** on B99

⌨ **Type** Target population

⌨ **Press** [tab] to move to the next field

⌨ **Type** =C98↵

🖱 **AutoFill** the formula from cell C99 across to E99.

However, whilst the total population was required above, this is not the case for the other columns in the table: this time it is the total population of babies who are available for checks or for immunisations. This figure will be smaller than the total population according to how many days it is from their birth date to today. For example, a baby born 3 weeks ago will not yet be ready for the 6-week check and is therefore not part of the population we are trying to reach.

In order to work out the total eligible population for F99 to K99 we must first set up a new column in L which will use a logical test to ensure that the population we seek is the one required. Effectively, we shall select from all the records those where the dates of birth are more than 42 days ago (i.e. 6 weeks) in order to provide the total required population. In logical terms we say:

'If today minus 42 days (i.e. 6 weeks) is greater than the birth date, place a '1' in the cell (the answer is true), otherwise place a '0' in the cell (the answer is false).'

To implement this in our sheet, we are going to use the columns on the right. First, we must remove any spurious formatting we placed there earlier in this chapter:

🖱 **Click** on the L in the column header

🖱 **Click** on Format to select the format menu

🖱 **Click** on Cells

🖱 **Click** on the Number tab

🖱 **Click** on 'All' from the Category list

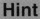 **Click** on 'General' from the list of format codes

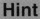 **Click** on ☐ OK ☐.

Now we can add our formulae:

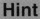 **Click** on L2

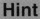 **Click** on *f* in the toolbar

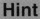 **Click** on 'Logical' in the list of function categories

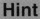 **Click** on 'IF' in the list of functions

 Click on ☐ OK ☐.

The dialog box is shown below:

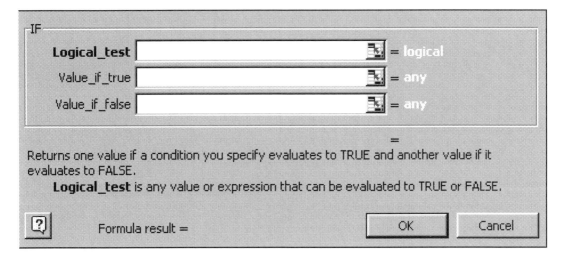

 Type TODAY()-42>$D2 in the logical test box (where the cursor is flashing).

 Press [tab].

Hint

This is the first example of the use of an absolute reference indicated by the '$'. This means that the column reference will not change as the formula is copied across a row of cells.

⌨ **Type** 1 in the value if true box then **Press** [tab].

⌨ **Type** 0 in the value if false box then **Press** [tab].

The completed version is shown below:

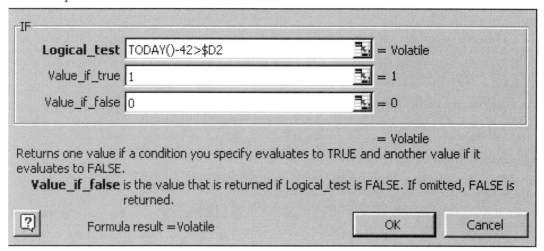

Once this dialog box is satisfactory:

🖰 **Click** on ⎡ OK ⎤.

The complete formula stored in cell L2 now reads:

=IF(TODAY()-42>$D2,1,0)

This is Excel's way of representing what is contained in the box. In the simplest possible terms, if the child is more than 6 weeks old, a '1' is placed in the cell, if not a '0' appears.

Hint

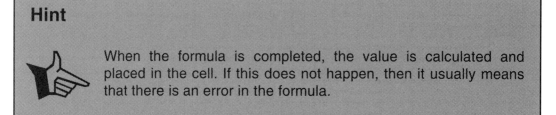

When the formula is completed, the value is calculated and placed in the cell. If this does not happen, then it usually means that there is an error in the formula.

🖰 **AutoFill** down the column to L97

🖰 **Click** on L98

🖰 **Click** on Σ

🖱 **Click** on ☑ or ⌨ **Press** ↵ to accept the formula.

This totals the column for you, and represents the maximum population available for the 6-week check today.

🖱 **AutoFill** the formula from L2 across to M2

🖱 **Double-click** on M2

⌨ Edit the cell from the keyboard so that the formula reads:
IF(TODAY()-$D2>62,1,0)

🖱 **AutoFill** the formula down the column to M14

🖱 **Click** on M97.

We will sum the column later using AutoFill. The total of this column represents the target population of children up to 2 months old.

Now repeat this process for columns N, O, P, Q placing:
IF(TODAY()-$D2>93,1,0) in cell N2, (*corresponds to 3 months ago*)
IF(TODAY()-$D2>124,1,0) in cell O2, (*corresponds to 4 months ago*)
IF(TODAY()-$D2>217,1,0) in cell P2, (*corresponds to 7 months ago*)
IF(TODAY()-$D2>372,1,0) in cell Q2, (*corresponds to 12 months ago*)
and then AutoFilling down to N97,O97,P97,Q97 respectively.

Finally, AutoFill across the summation formula in L98 as far as Q98 to calculate the respective populations.

Hint

If you use AutoFill to copy the formula across from N2 to Q2, then edit the formulae to their appropriate values, then highlight the cells N2 to Q2, you can AutoFill the whole row down to fill the entire range of cells.

To transfer these values to the main table

The final stage is to transfer these values back to the main table. The value for the target population calculated in cell L98 is needed in F99.

To accomplish this:

🖱 **Click** on F99

⌨ **Type** = L98.

Similarly, the value for the second target population in M98 is needed in G99. This can be readily accomplished using AutoFill:

🖱 **Click** on F99

🖱 **AutoFill** from F99 across to K99.

Now that we have target populations and the number of infants reached, we can work out the percentage reached using a simple division sum:

🖱 **Click** on B100

⌨ **Type** Percentage reached ↵

🖱 **Click** on C100

⌨ **Type** =C98/C99

🖱 **AutoFill** to copy the formula across to K100.

With the cells still highlighted, we can change the format to a percentage:

🖱 **Click** on Format to select the format menu

🖱 **Click** on Cells

🖱 **Click** on the Number tab

🖱 **Click** on Percentage from the Category list

🖱 **Click** twice on   to reduce the number of decimal places

🖱 **Click** on OK .

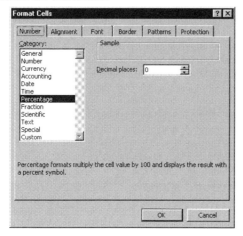

Using compound formulae to simplify (!) calculations

Health warning

The next section is not for the faint-hearted! Further, it will simply enable you to do what you've already done in a more elegant and compact way – so you can miss it out without significant loss.

If you are in any doubt, then miss it out and come back later

The previous solution used elementary steps to arrive at a performance measure but we can combine these elementary steps to produce a more compact sheet. The problem is that the sheet becomes even less comprehensible. If you still wish to proceed, then pour yourself an extra strong cup of tea, and here goes.

To do this we can use a compound statement. First, let's delete the formulae in columns L to Q:

🖰 **Highlight** L2 to Q98

⌨ **Press** [Del]

🖰 **Double-click** on F99

⌨ **Type** =SUM(IF(TODAY()-$D2:$D97>42,1,0)).

Health warning

Do **not** hit the ↵ key! Instead, read the next paragraph before proceeding

We are now going to make use of a compound statement. A compound statement combines two steps in one. Previously, we have used an IF statement for each record and then summed the whole column. Here we combine the two steps into one command. Remember to tell Excel that it is a compound statement by pressing [Ctrl] and [⇧] and ↵ instead of simply↵. This must be repeated for any edits or changes. This statement also makes use of the idea of an array. An array is a group of cells to which we can apply an instruction. Thus in this case, our array is D2:D14. We have actually already used arrays in conjunction with the SUM() command alone, without drawing attention to them.

⌨ **Hold down** [Ctrl]and [⇧] and **Press.**↵

🖱 **AutoFill** the formulae across to K15

🖱 **Double-click** on G15

⌨ Change the figure 42 to 62 by typing at the keyboard

⌨ **Hold down** [Ctrl]and [⇧] and **Press** ↵

🖱 **Double-click** on H15

⌨ Change the figure 42 to 93 by typing at the keyboard

⌨ **Hold down** [Ctrl]and [⇧] and **Press** ↵

🖱 **Double-click** on I15

⌨ Change the figure 42 to 124 by typing at the keyboard

⌨ **Hold down** [Ctrl]and [⇧] and **Press** ↵

🖱 **Double-click** on J15

⌨ Change the figure 42 to 217 by typing at the keyboard

⌨ **Hold down** [Ctrl]and [⇧] and **Press** ↵

🖱 **Double-click** on K15

⌨ Change the figure 42 to 372 by typing at the keyboard

⌨ Hold down [Ctrl]and [⇧] and Press ↵.

The result should be the same as before.

Hint

The faint-hearted, i.e. the kind of people who see no fun in climbing a mountain in a raging blizzard when they saw it on a sunny day yesterday, may re-enter here.

Keeping notes

The information shown in an individual cell may not tell the whole tale. It is possible to add notes to each of the cells in the sheet to provide more explanation:

 🖰 **Click** on a blank cell in Column G relating to the first triple

 🖰 **Click** on Insert in the menu bar

 🖰 **Click** on Comment.

Excel opens a box for a comment and adds the user's name:

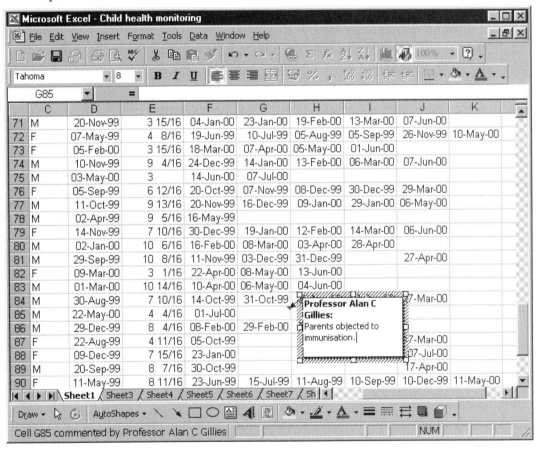

 ⌨ **Type** a note, e.g. spoke to parent: objected to immunisation.

 🖰 **Click** on the main sheet to save the comment and store it in the cell, denoted by a red triangle.

To open a comment, simply move the pointer over the relevant cell and the comment appears.

Very often, the same note may crop up in different cells. For example, in this case, we may wish to include the same note in cells H12 and I12. To do this:

🖱 **Click** on the cell with the note attached

🖱 **Click** on 📋

🖱 **Click** on another blank cell

🖱 **Click** on <u>E</u>dit in the menu bar

🖱 **Click** on Paste <u>S</u>pecial

🖱 **Click** on <u>C</u>omments from the resulting dialog box

🖱 **Click** on ⟨ OK ⟩

🖱 **Press** [Esc] to remove outline marquee.

The note is now attached to each of the blank cells and the note indicator should appear in both of them.

Hint

Note that in these days of multimedia, Excel will even store spoken notes!

In those immortal words: 'investigation of this matter is left as an exercise for the reader'.

Adding the date and time to a sheet

It is sometimes useful to show when a sheet was actually produced and printed. We will add the date and time to the sheet:

🖱 **Click** on A100

🖱 **Click** on *f*ₓ

🖱 **Click** on Date & Time in the list of function categories

🖱 **Click** on 'NOW()' (gives today's date) from the list of functions

🖱 **Click** on ⟨ OK ⟩.

This gives today's date and time.

This is automatically updated so any printouts will provide an automatic date and time stamp.

Exercise

Using the techniques learnt in the opening scenario, plot a 3-D column chart based upon the performance indicators obtained in this section to show the percentage of the target population reached for each of the following:

- 6-week check
- Triple 1
- Triple 2
- Triple 3
- 7-month check
- 12-month MMR.

Governance scenario 3

Outpatient orthopaedic clinic in secondary care

In this chapter

This chapter will tell you how to:

- analyse results from a patient survey

- construct a frequency distribution table

- construct a frequency distribution chart

- use a chi-squared test to evaluate relationships between variables

 manage date and time data in Excel

 use compound statements

 combine logical and numerical formulae

 manage multiple worksheets within a workbook

 use the CHITEST() function.

The scenario

The outpatient orthopaedic clinic at Knapford General Hospital is extremely busy. There have been reports of patients experiencing delays before seeing the doctor. As part of the clinical governance effort, an audit has been established to investigate the extent of the problem, and patients' perception of it.

Patients attending the clinic during the first 6 months of 1992 were asked to fill in a simple questionnaire. The questionnaire was given out to patients on arrival at the clinic and they were given the opportunity to return the form at the end of their visit. During this time, 1054 patients visited the clinic. Of these, 762 returned the forms, of which 733 were suitable for analysis.

The survey focused upon the patient experience before entering the consulting room. The audit asked the patients for the length of time between their appointment time and the actual time that they got to see the doctor. The survey also asked patients for their perceptions of the experience.
The survey targets particularly children and their parents. Thus, child patients are identified and their parents' responses analysed separately. 257 of the 762 patients in the survey were in this category.

The aim of the audit is stated as:

'To investigate the patients' view of care in an outpatient clinic'.

If we pursue this further, we can define a specific set of objectives which arise from this overall aim, i.e.:

1 to determine waiting times between referral and appointment
2 to determine waiting times within the clinic to see a doctor
3 to determine patient satisfaction with waiting times
4 to determine patient satisfaction with the waiting environment.

Each of these objectives then defines the data and analysis requirements of the audit.

To meet objective 1, it is necessary to collect two pieces of data for each patient: the date of a request for an appointment and the date of the actual appointment. These are date fields and may be gathered from patient records.

Similarly, in order to establish waiting times in the clinic itself, it is necessary to monitor the time of appointment and the actual time at which seen by the doctor. This cannot be carried out retrospectively from records as it is not usual to record the time at which the patient was actually seen. This data would have to be recorded separately.

The data could be gathered from patients, since a patient questionnaire is required to address objective 3. To satisfy objective 3, it would be necessary to elicit patient views from a question such as the first one shown below.

How satisfied were you with the length of time you had to wait to see a doctor at the clinic?

1 Very satisfied   [ ]
2 Quite satisfied   [ ]
3 No strong feelings   [ ]
4 Quite dissatisfied   [ ]
5 Very dissatisfied   [ ]

How did you feel about the waiting area at the clinic?

1 Very satisfied   [ ]
2 Quite satisfied   [ ]
3 No strong feelings   [ ]
4 Quite dissatisfied   [ ]
5 Very dissatisfied   [ ]

This could be recorded as a numerical satisfaction measure ranging from +2 to -2. In order to meet objective 4, a similar approach could be adopted, based around a question such as the second one above.

It is also necessary to decide whether there is any subsidiary data required to break down the groups further. For example, the audit introduction identifies child patients as a priority group within the study. Thus, it is necessary to include a data field for a child patient, stored as a 'Yes/No' field, allowing the overall results to be broken down in this way.

The data collected by the survey is stored in the sheet 'outpatient survey.xls'.

🖰 **Open** outpatient survey.xls.

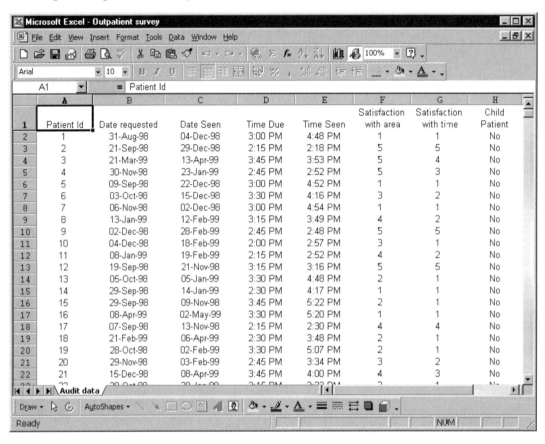

The sheet contains eight columns of data for 733 patients.

The table below lists the data gathered, the format in which it is stored, and where the data was gathered from.

As noted previously, it is good practice to leave our original dataset intact. To do this, we simply copy the whole sheet. This is a reprise of one you did earlier in Scenario 1:

🖰 **Click** on Edit in the menu bar

🖰 **Click** on Move or Copy Sheet in the Edit menu

🖰 **Click** on (move to end)

Column	Header	Data format	Data stored
A	Patient Id	Number (integer)	Sequential patient id (assigned in sheet)
B	Date requested	Date (dd-mm-yy)	Date appointment requested (from patient records)
C	Date seen	Date (dd-mm-yy)	Date of actual appointment (from patient records)
D	Time due	Time (12 hour)	Time due to be seen (from clinic records)
E	Time seen	Time (12 hour)	Time actually seen (from clinic records)
F	Satisfaction with area	Number (integer)	Rating: 1–5 (from patient survey)
G	Satisfaction with time	Number (integer)	Rating: 1–5 (from patient survey)
H	Child patient	Text (yes/no)	Whether patient is child (from patient records)

🖱 **Click** on <u>C</u>reate a copy

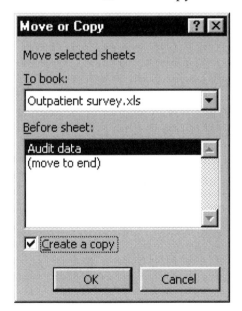

🖱 **Click** on ⬛ OK .

This creates a copy of the whole sheet.

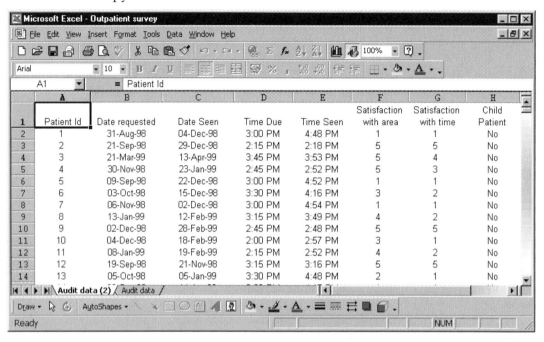

🖱 **Double-click** on the Audit data (2) tab to rename it.

⌨ **Type** Data Analysis.

The other thing we can do is to protect a sheet. To do this:

🖱 **Click** on <u>T</u>ools in the menu bar

🖱 **Click** on <u>P</u>rotection in the <u>T</u>ools menu

🖱 **Click** on <u>P</u>rotect Sheet in the sub-menu

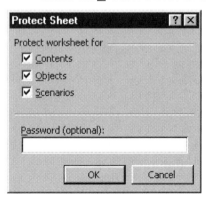

🖱 **Click** on OK .

Health warning

Since the sheet protection is left as an exercise for the reader, the basic data sheet as provided is unprotected. Therefore, please ensure that the protection is carried out properly.

You have been warned!

Hint

Excel treats dates and times as numbers and a variety of formats are available. However, regardless of the format used to display, Excel stores all dates as numbers, hidden from the user if the date format is used.

To display the actual number that Excel uses to store a date, select the cells that contain the date or time:

🖱 **Click** on Format in the menu bar

🖱 **Click** on Cells in the Format menu

🖱 **Click** on the Number tab

🖱 **Click** on General in the Category box.

In Excel, days are numbered from the beginning of the century; the date January 1, 1900 is represented as 1. See below for the implications of storing and manipulating times.

N.B. If Excel appears to misbehave, then get someone to check how your software is set up. It is possible to set up Excel in other ways.

The first factor to investigate is the waiting time for patients to receive a clinic appointment. As this is a multi-factor study we will use a distinct sheet to analyse each factor. We will therefore create a frequency distribution table in Sheet 1. The first task is to establish the waiting time in days. The number of days' waiting time is simply the difference between the two dates:

🖰 **Click** on the tab labelled 'Sheet1'.

At cell A1:

⌨ **Type** waiting times↵.

At cell A2, enter the following formula:

⌨ **Type** =

🖰 **Click** on the tab labelled 'Data Analysis'

🖰 **Click** on C2

⌨ **Type** -

🖰 **Click** on B2

⌨ **Press** ↵

The formula in Sheet1, cell A2 should now read:

='Data Analysis'!C2-'Data Analysis'!B2, and the correct answer is 95 (the time in days for the first patient between the appointment request and the appointment itself).

Now:

🖰 **AutoFill** down from A2 to A734 in Sheet1.

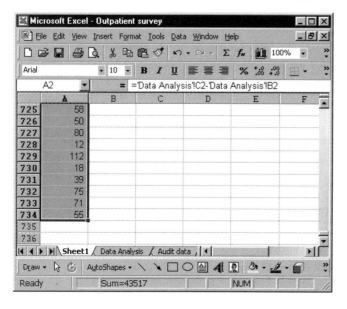

⟋ **Press** [Ctrl] and [Home] to get back to the top.

First, we need to examine this data. To do this, we can use a useful bit of Excel called the Analysis Toolpak Add-In. The good news is that it's full of good stuff. The bad news is that it's probably not installed on your system. No problem! See below.

Health warning

The Analysis ToolPak may not be installed on your machine. To check:

⟋ **Click** on Tools in the menu bar.

If the option Data Analysis is on the menu, then you're OK; if not, then read the following Hint.

Remember that Excel may not show you the whole menu at first, wait until the full menu appears.

Hint

To install the Analysis ToolPak, if not already there:

⟋ **Click** on Tools in the menu bar

⟋ **Click** on Add-ins on the Tools menu

⟋ **Click** on Analysis ToolPak from the list of Add-ins available

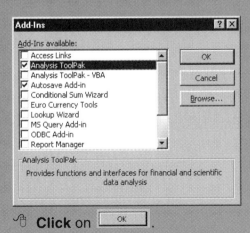

⟋ **Click** on OK .

🖰 **Click** on Tools in the bar

🖰 **Click** on Data Analysis in the Tools menu

🖰 **Click** on Descriptive Statistics in the list of tools available

🖰 **Click** on ⬜ OK ⬜

⌨ **Type** A1:A734 in the Input Range box

🖰 **Click** on Labels in First Row

🖰 **Click** on Output Range

⌨ **Type** C1:A734 in the Output Range box

🖰 **Click** on Summary Statistics.

The options selected should look like the one below:

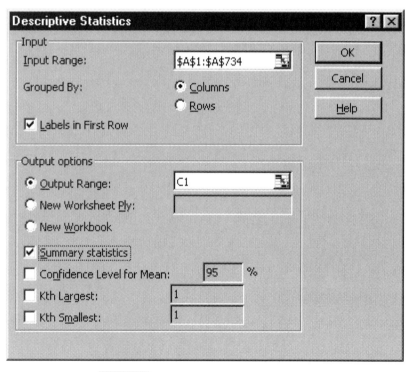

🖰 **Click** on ⬜ OK ⬜.

The result (after a little bit of optional cosmetic tidying, font change plus column width change) should look like the one below.

Summary statistics calculates in one go:

- Mean
- Median
- Standard deviation
- Kurtosis
- Range
- Maximum
- Count
- Standard error
- Mode
- Sample variance
- Skewness
- Minimum
- Sum.

Remember the principle of constructive laziness!

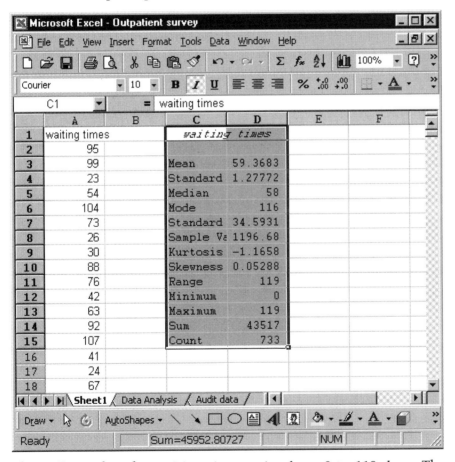

This tells us that the waiting time varies from 0 to 119 days. The mean waiting time is 59 days, and the median is 58. However, the distribution is unlikely to be normal with a mode of 119. What we really need is a picture to see what is going on.

For this we first construct a frequency distribution table, then a frequency distribution chart:

🖰 **Click** on C17

⌨ **Type** Frequency distribution↵

⌨ **Type** Range

⌨ **Press** [Tab]

⌨ **Type** Frequency

⌨ **Press** ↵

⌨ **Press** [Left arrow]

⌨ **Type** 0 to 11↵   in cell C19

⌨ **Type** 12 to 23↵   in cell C20

⌨ **Type** 24 to 35↵   in cell C21

⌨ **Type** 36 to 47↵   in cell C22

⌨ **Type** 48 to 63↵   in cell C23

⌨ **Type** 64 to 71↵   in cell C24

⌨ **Type** 72 to 83↵   in cell C25

⌨ **Type** 84 to 95↵   in cell C26

⌨ **Type** 96 to 107↵   in cell C27

⌨ **Type** 108 to 119↵   in cell C28

🖰 **Click** on D19.

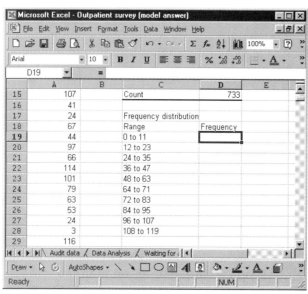

Now to construct our frequency distribution table.

In D19, we need to count the number of patients waiting less than 12 days. We can do this using a simple function:

🖱 **Click** on 𝑓𝑥

🖱 **Click** on Statistical in the Function category list

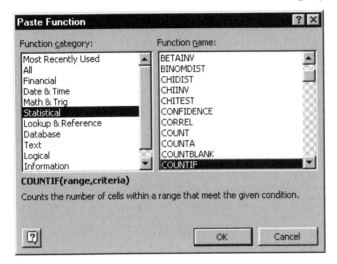

🖱 **Click** on the scroll bar bottom arrow until COUNTIF is visible

🖱 **Click** on COUNTIF

⌨ **Type** A$2:A$734

⌨ **Press** [Tab]

⌨ **Type** <12

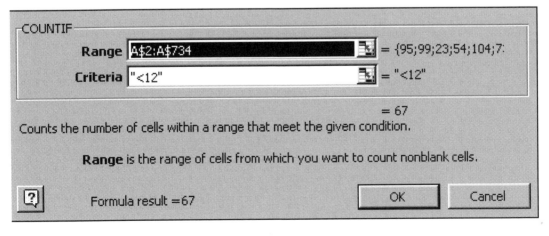

⌨ Press ↵.

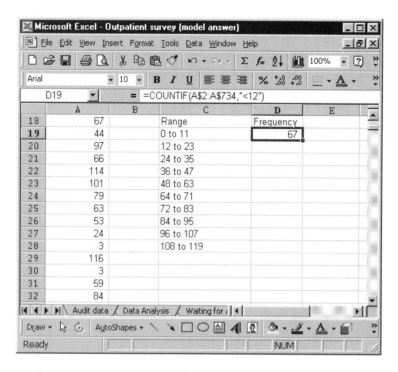

Unfortunately, COUNTIF has some limitations in use which mean that if we want to use it for the later rows, we must use it to calculate a cumulative frequency, then subtract the previous cumulative frequency.

To see how this works:

🖱 **Autofill** the formula in D19 down to D20

🖱 **Click** on D20

🖱 **Highlight** 12   in the formula

⌨ **Type** 24   to replace it

⌨ **Press** [End]

⌨ **Type** -D19

⌨ **Press** ↵

🖱 **Click** on D20

🖱 **Autofill** the formula in D20 down to D21

🖱 **Click** on D21

🖱 **Highlight** 24   in the formula

⌨ **Type** 36   to replace it

🖱 **Highlight** D19   in the formula

⌨️ **Type** sum(D$19:D20)   to replace it

⌨️ **Press** ↵

🖱️ **Click** on D21

🖱️ **Autofill** the formula in D21 down to D28

🖱️ **Click** on D22.

Now replace the 36 in each formulae in E22 to E28 as above to read 48, 60, 72, 84, 96, 108, 120 respectively.

The final table should look like the one below.

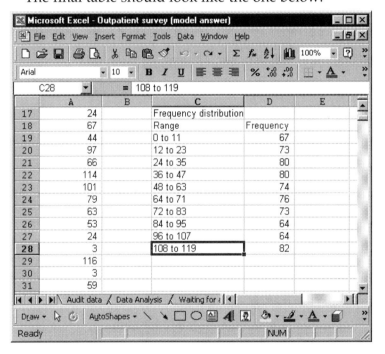

Exercise

The production of a frequency distribution chart from this table in the form of a simple 3-D column chart is a revision of previous work carried out in Scenarios 1 and 2. It is therefore left as an exercise for the reader.

A model answer is shown overleaf.

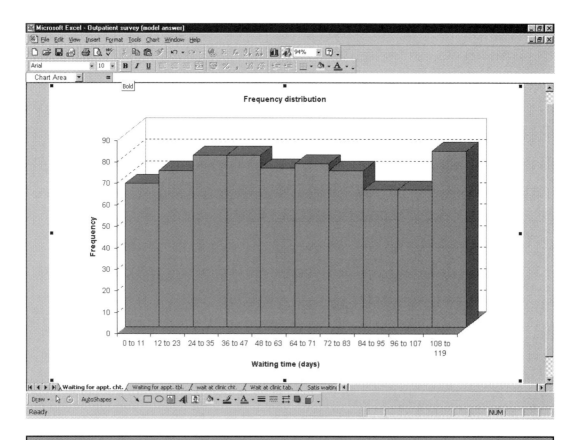

Health warning

In this example, the waiting time bands were deliberately chosen so that they were equal.

In other situations, this may not be the case. For example, WHO defines standard age ranges for its statistics that are not equal.

In such cases, the width of the bars of the chart should reflect the width of the bands used to group the data. To the best of my knowledge this is not possible within Excel. You have three choices:

1 Prove me wrong
2 Publish your chart with a cautionary warning
3 Export your data to a specialist statistics package.

My best fudge is given on the website!

Before we do more analysis, it is helpful to label the sheets in our book:

🖑 **Double-click** on the tab labelled 'Chart1' containing the frequency distribution chart

⌨ **Type** Waiting for appt. cht

🖑 **Double-click** on the tab labelled 'Sheet1' containing the frequency distribution table

⌨ **Type** Waiting for appt. tbl.

Now we want to repeat the previous analysis for waiting times at the clinic itself.

For this we need to consider how Excel stores time. See the next hint box. Most of the time we choose how to format our times, as either 12 or 24-hour clock, then Excel does the rest. However, we need to think a bit harder to do calculations on times.

Let's set up our analysis in Sheet 2. First rename it 'Wait at clinic tbl':

🖑 **Double-click** on the tab labelled 'Sheet2' (it should be blank!)

⌨ **Type** Wait at clinic tbl.

Now to the analysis itself. The first task is to establish the waiting time in minutes.

Hint

Remember, Excel treats dates and times as numbers. A single number is used to store a date and time.

To display the actual number that Excel uses to store a time, select the cells that contain the time:

🖑 **Click** on Format in the menu bar

🖑 **Click** on Cells in the Format menu

🖑 **Click** on the Number tab

🖑 **Click** on General in the Category box.

In Excel, each day is counted as 1. The decimal part of the number represents the time. In each day there are 1440 minutes, so each minute is equivalent to 1/1440, or 6.944×10^{-4}.

Thus, the following numbers are used to represent times, if no date is attached:

24-hour	12-hour	General
12:00	12:00 PM	0.5
13:00	1:00 PM	0.541667
13:30	1:30 PM	0.5625
13:45	1:45 PM	0.572917
13:51	1:51 PM	0.577083

2:30 pm on Aug 21 1999 would be represented by the number 36393.1041666667!

In simple terms, to work out the difference between two times in minutes, take the difference between the cells and multiply it by 1440, the number of minutes in a day.

The number of minutes waiting time is given as the difference between the two times, multiplied by 1440, as explained above.

At cell A1:

⌨ **Type** waiting times↵.

At cell A2, enter the following formula:

⌨ **Type** =(

🖱 **Click** on the tab labelled 'Data Analysis'

🖱 **Click** on E2

⌨ **Type** -

🖱 **Click** on D2

⌨ **Type**)*1440

⌨ **Press** ↵.

The formula in Sheet1, cell A2 should now read

=('Data Analysis'!E2-'Data Analysis'!D2)*1440,
and the correct answer is 108.963.

(This is the time in minutes for the first patient between the time seen and the time of the appointment itself.)

Hint

It's not an integer, because Excel stores minutes as parts of days.

Let's tidy up the format to give whole numbers:

- 🖰 **Highlight** Column A
- 🖰 **Click** on Format in the menu bar
- 🖰 **Click** on Cells in the Format menu
- 🖰 **Click** on the Number tab
- 🖰 **Click** on Number in the Category box
- 🖰 **Click** on ▾ twice to reduce the number of Decimal places to 0
- 🖰 **AutoFill** down from A2 to A734

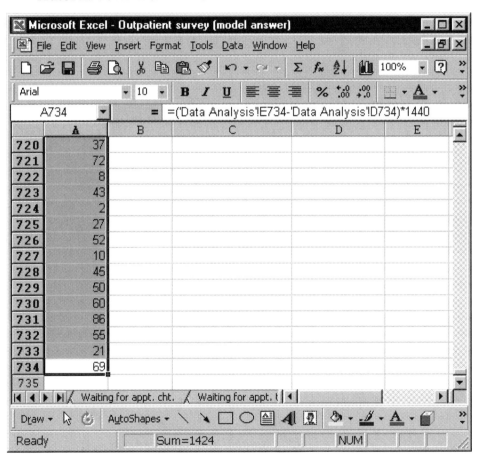

⌨ **Press** [Ctrl] and [Home] to get back to the top.

Next we examine this data using the Analysis Toolpak again:

- 🖰 **Click** on Tools in the bar

🖰 **Click** on <u>D</u>ata Analysis in the <u>T</u>ools menu

🖰 **Click** on Descriptive Statistics in the list of tools available

🖰 **Click** on [OK]

⌨ **Type** A1:A734 in the <u>I</u>nput Range box

🖰 **Click** on <u>L</u>abels in First Row

🖰 **Click** on Output Range

⌨ **Type** C1:A734 in the <u>O</u>utput Range box

🖰 **Click** on <u>S</u>ummary Statistics.

The options selected should look the same as last time:

🖰 **Click** on [OK].

The result (after a little bit of optional cosmetic tidying, font change plus column width change) should look like the one below:

	A	B	C	D	E
1	waiting time		*Column1*		
2	109				
3	3		Mean	45.88891483	
4	8		Standard Error	1.190527816	
5	8		Median	40.70440867	
6	113		Mode	#N/A	
7	47		Standard Deviation	32.23231765	
8	115		Sample Variance	1038.922301	
9	34		Kurtosis	-0.570835359	
10	4		Skewness	0.61728155	
11	57		Range	119.5555386	
12	37		Minimum	0.147349398	
13	1		Maximum	119.702888	
14	79		Sum	33636.57457	
15	107		Count	733	
16	97				

Microsoft Excel - Outpatient survey (model answer)

File Edit View Insert Format Tools Data Window Help

Arial 10 B I U

A1 = waiting time

Waiting for appt. cht. Waiting for appt. t

Draw AutoShapes

Ready NUM

This tells us that the waiting time varies from 0 to 2 hours. The mean waiting time is 46 minutes, and the median is 41. However, there is no mode defined.

Note that the Analysis Toolpak works on the underlying figures, not the whole numbers presented in the sheet. This is why there is no mode calculated.

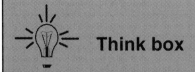

Think box

How can we convert the actual numbers?

See the Hints section on the website for an answer if you get stuck.

Now we will first construct the frequency distribution table, then the frequency distribution chart:

🖰 **Click** on C17

⌨ **Type** Frequency distribution ↵

⌨ **Type** Range

⌨ **Press** [Tab]

⌨ **Type** Frequency

⌨ **Press** ↵

⌨ **Press** [Left arrow]

⌨ **Type** 0 to 11↵   in cell C19

⌨ **Type** 12 to 23↵   in cell C20

⌨ **Type** 24 to 35↵   in cell C21

⌨ **Type** 36 to 47↵   in cell C22

⌨ **Type** 48 to 63↵   in cell C23

⌨ **Type** 64 to 71↵   in cell C24

⌨ **Type** 72 to 83↵   in cell C25

⌨ **Type** 84 to 95↵   in cell C26

⌨ **Type** 96 to 107↵   in cell C27

⌨ **Type** 108 to 119↵   in cell C28

🖰 **Click** on D19.

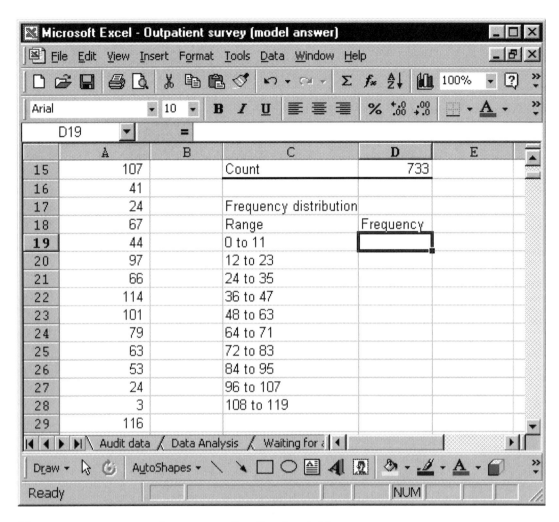

Now to construct our frequency distribution table.

In D19, we need to count the number of patients waiting less than 12 minutes. We can do this using a simple function:

🖰 **Click** on 𝑓ₓ

🖰 **Click** on Statistical in the Function category list

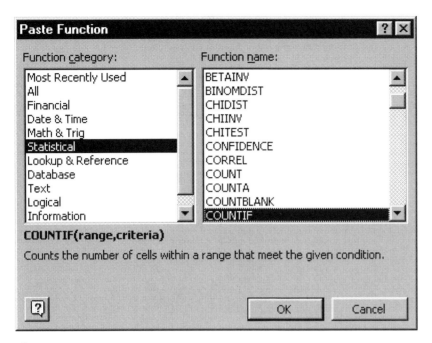

🖑 **Click** on the scroll bar bottom arrow until COUNTIF is visible

🖑 **Click** on COUNTIF

⌨ **Type** A$2:A$734

⌨ **Press** [Tab]

⌨ **Type** <12

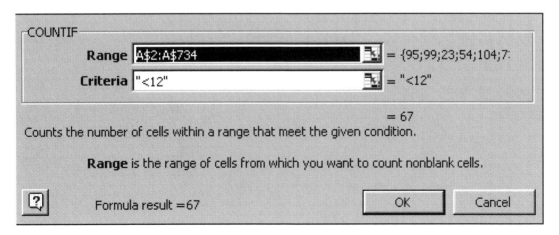

⌨ **Press** ↵.

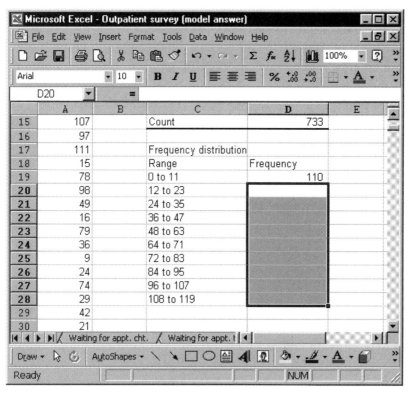

To complete the rest of the table:

🖱 **Autofill** the formula in D19 down to D20

🖱 **Click** on D20

🖱 **Highlight** 12   in the formula

⌨ **Type** 24   to replace it

⌨ **Press** [End]

⌨ **Type** –D19

⌨ **Press** ⏎

🖱 **Click** on D20

🖱 **Autofill** the formula in D20 down to D21

🖱 **Click** on D21

🖱 **Highlight** 24   in the formula

⌨ **Type** 36   to replace it

🖱 **Highlight** D19   in the formula

⌨ **Type** sum(D$19:D20)   to replace it

⌨ **Press** ↵

🖰 **Click** on D21

🖰 **Autofill** the formula in D21 down to D28

🖰 **Click** on D22

Now replace the 36 in each formulae in E22 to E28 as above to read 48, 60, 72, 84, 96, 108, 120 respectively.

The final table should look like the one below:

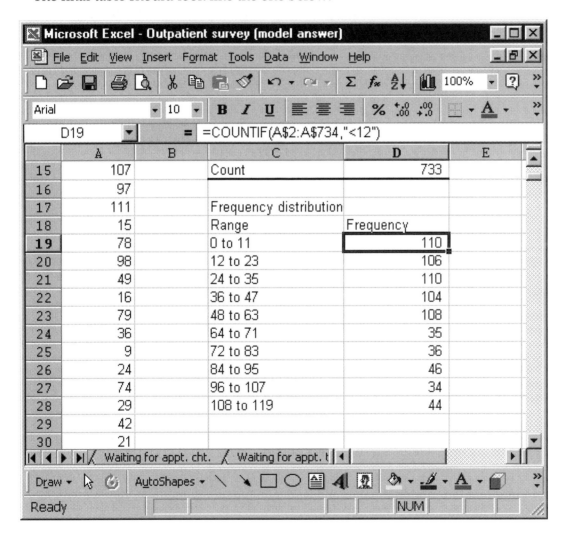

Exercise

The production of a frequency distribution chart from this table in the form of a simple 3-D column chart is a revision of previous work carried out in Scenarios 1 and 2. It is therefore left as an exercise for the reader.

A model answer is shown below.

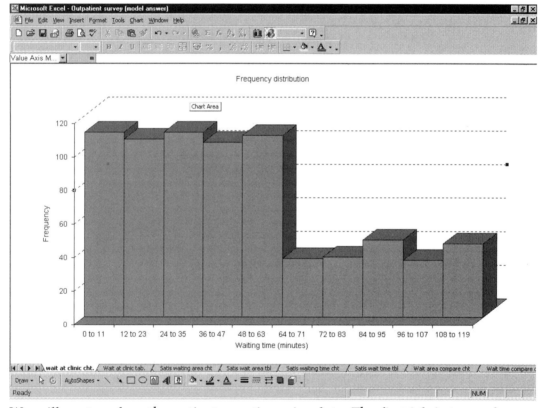

We will next analyse the patient questionnaire data. The first job is to produce a frequency distribution table and chart in the same manner as above.

The first step is identical, so for our next exercise:

Exercise

Produce descriptive statistics for the 'satisfaction with waiting area' data in the manner described above.

> **Small hint**: the formula required in cell A2 of the sheet used to analyse the data should read ='Data Analysis'!F2

The finished sheet should look like the one below.

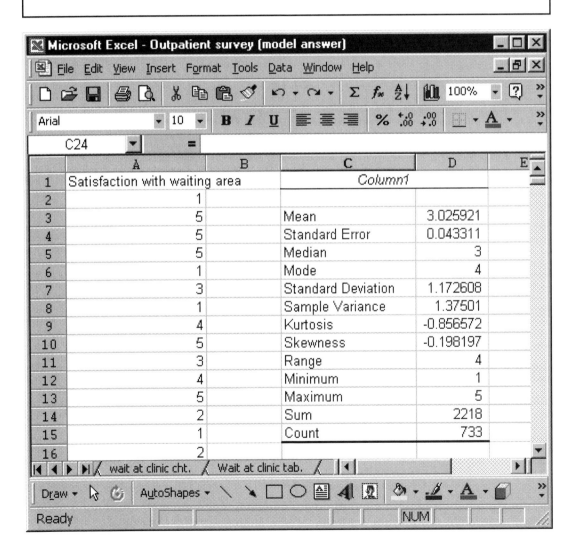

	A	B	C	D	E
1	Satisfaction with waiting area		*Column1*		
2	1				
3	5		Mean	3.025921	
4	5		Standard Error	0.043311	
5	5		Median	3	
6	1		Mode	4	
7	3		Standard Deviation	1.172608	
8	1		Sample Variance	1.37501	
9	4		Kurtosis	-0.856572	
10	5		Skewness	-0.198197	
11	3		Range	4	
12	4		Minimum	1	
13	5		Maximum	5	
14	2		Sum	2218	
15	1		Count	733	
16	2				

Our frequency distribution table is simpler this time:

🖑 **Click** on C17

⌨ **Type** Frequency distribution↵

⌨ **Type** Range

⌨ **Press** [Tab]

⌨ **Type** Frequency

⌨ **Press** ↵

⌨ **Press** [Left arrow]

⌨ **Type** 1

⌨ **Press** ↵

⌨ **Type** =C19+1

🖑 **AutoFill** down to C23.

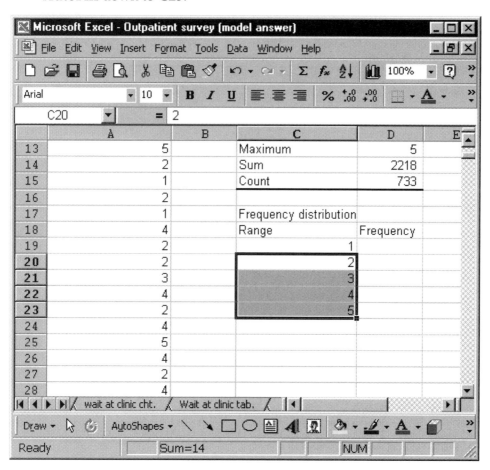

The frequency calculation is a simpler use of the COUNTIF() function:

- ↗ **Click** on D19

- ↗ **Click** on **f_***

- ↗ **Click** on Statistical in the Function category list if the COUNTIF function is not visible in the Most Recently Used category

- ↗ **Click** on the scroll bar bottom arrow until COUNTIF is visible

- ↗ **Click** on COUNTIF

- ⌨ **Type** A2:A734

- ⌨ **Press** [Tab]

- ⌨ **Type** C19

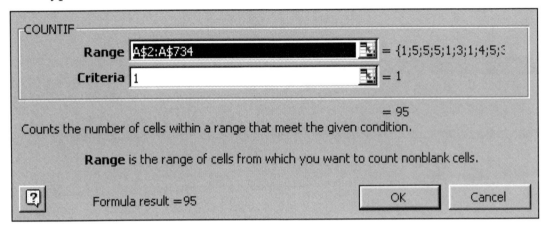

- ⌨ **Press** ↵

- ↗ **AutoFill** down to C23.

The final result is given below.

Exercise

The production of a frequency distribution chart from this table in the form of a simple 3-D column chart is a revision of previous work carried out in Scenarios 1 and 2. It is therefore left as an exercise for the reader.

A model answer is shown overleaf.

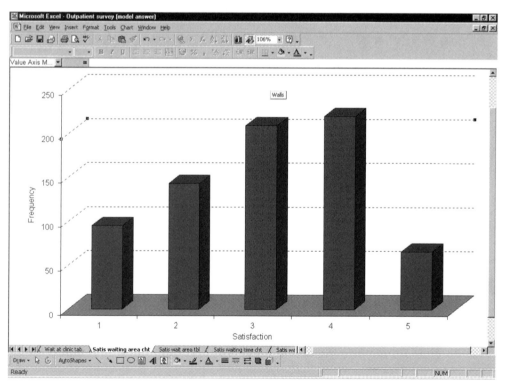

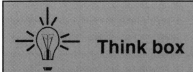

Think box

How can we convert the numbers on the x axis to the actual responses? The final graph might look like the one below.

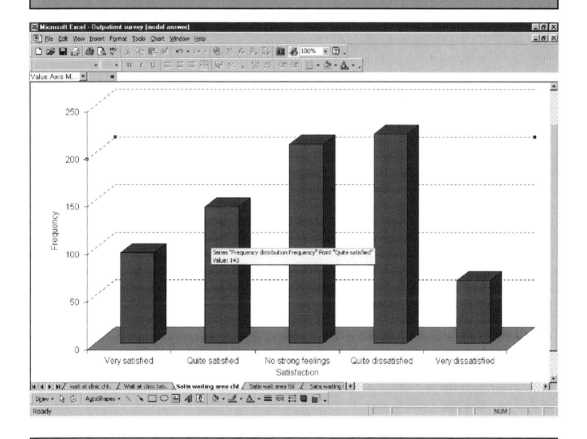

Exercise

The analysis of the satisfaction data for the waiting time is identical in almost every detail. Model answers for the data sheet and chart follow.

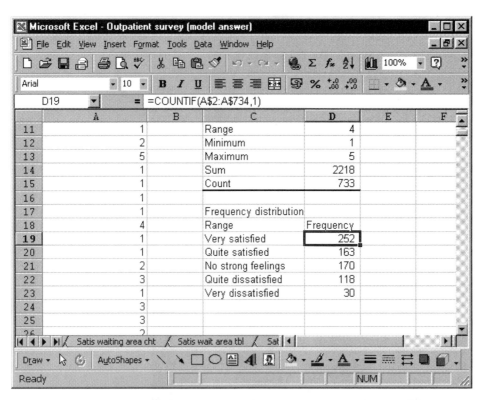

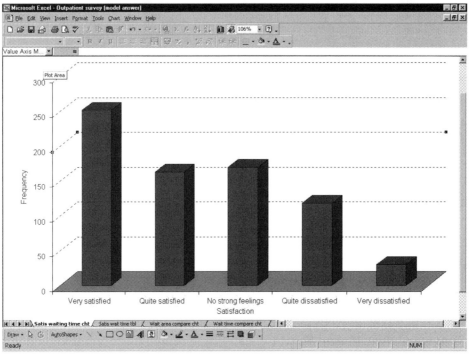

Health warning

The following hint is not recommended for beginners, and is therefore in outline only. If you don't feel confident to work it out from these instructions, then come back later and move on for now.

The next step is to compare the results for child patients with those of adults. We

Hint

There is a quick way to do this.

1 Make copies of the two most recent sheets:

🖰 **Highlight** the sheets 'satis wait area tbl' and 'satis wait area cht' using the tabs at the bottom and the [Ctrl] key to select the second whilst keeping the first selected

🖰 **Click** on Edit

🖰 **Click** on Move or copy sheet

🖰 **Click** on (move to end) in the Before sheet box

🖰 **Click** in the Create a copy box

🖰 **Click** on ⬜ OK ⬜.

2 Rename the copied sheets:

🖰 **Double-click** on the tabs at the bottom of the relevant sheets.

3 Change the references to 'area' to 'time'.

4 Change the formula in A2 to read
='Data Analysis'!G2.

5 🖰 **AutoFill** the new formula down to A734.

The end result should be the same

do this by conducting a stratified frequency distribution table:

- ⌐ **Click** on the tab at the bottom marked 'Sheet4' – this should be blank
- ⌐ **Click** on C1
- ▦ **Type** Waiting area
- ▦ **Press** [Tab] twice
- ▦ **Type** Waiting time
- ⌐ **Click** on C1
- ▦ **Type** Adults
- ▦ **Press** [Tab]
- ▦ **Type** Children
- ▦ **Press** [Tab]
- ⌐ **Autofill** labels across to F2
- ⌐ **Click** on A3
- ▦ **Type** Very satisfied
- ▦ **Press** ↵
- ▦ **Type** Quite satisfied
- ▦ **Press** ↵
- ▦ **Type** No strong feelings
- ▦ **Press** ↵
- ▦ **Type** Quite dissatisfied
- ▦ **Press** ↵
- ▦ **Type** Very dissatisfied
- ▦ **Press** ↵
- ⌐ **Click** on B3
- ▦ **Type** 1
- ▦ **Press** ↵
- ▦ **Type** =B3+1
- ⌐ **Autofill** labels down to B7.

The text entered should look like the one below:

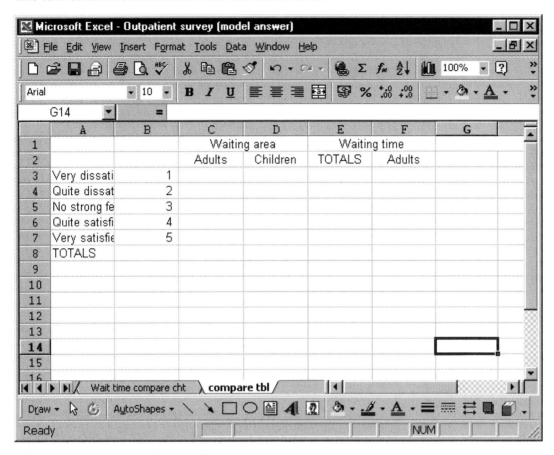

The next steps are to format the text:

🖱 **Highlight** Columns A and B

🖱 **Double-click** on the dividing line between the headers to Columns B and C to resize the columns to best fit their data

🖱 **Highlight** C1 and D1

🖱 **Click** on 🔲 to centre the heading across the two columns

🖱 **Highlight** E1 and F1

🖱 **Click** on 🔲 to centre the heading across the two columns.

The sheet should now look a bit tidier:

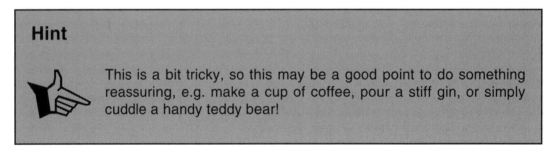

Now we need to calculate how many adult patients were very dissatisfied with the waiting area.

Hint

This is a bit tricky, so this may be a good point to do something reassuring, e.g. make a cup of coffee, pour a stiff gin, or simply cuddle a handy teddy bear!

The way that we do it is as follows:

If a patient is very dissatisfied (Column F=1), then we check to see if they are an adult (Column H=no). If both of these conditions are met, then we assign that patient a 1; if not, then we assign them a 0. When we have checked every patient, we tot up the 1s, by adding up the column.

In Excel speak, it looks like this:

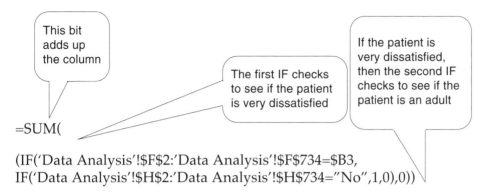

=SUM(

(IF('Data Analysis'!$F$2:'Data Analysis'!$F$734=$B3,
IF('Data Analysis'!$H$2:'Data Analysis'!$H$734="No",1,0),0))

To enter the formula in the sheet:

🖰 **Click** on C3

⌨ **Type** =SUM(IF('Data Analysis'!$F$2:'Data Analysis'!$F$734=$B3, IF('Data Analysis'!$H$2:'Data Analysis'!$H$734="No",1,0),0))

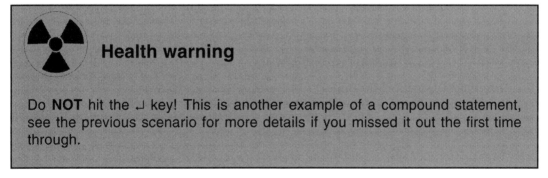

Health warning

Do **NOT** hit the ↵ key! This is another example of a compound statement, see the previous scenario for more details if you missed it out the first time through.

⌨ **Press** [Ctrl] and [Shift] and ↵ together to accept the compound formula.

The answer is 47. To make up for all this effort, to fill in the rest of this column:

🖰 **AutoFill** the formula down to C7.

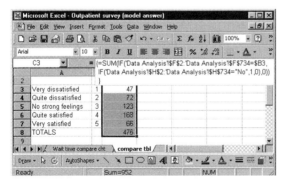

To save ourselves some more effort, we will AutoFill the formula across the top row and edit as appropriate:

🖑 **AutoFill** the formula across to F3

🖑 **Click** on D3

⌨ **Edit** the formula by replacing 'No' with 'Yes'.

The corrected formula should read:

=SUM(IF('Data Analysis'!$F$2:'Data Analysis'!$F$734=$B3, IF('Data Analysis' !$H$2:'Data Analysis'!$H$734="Yes",1,0),0))

⌨ **Press** [Ctrl] and [Shift] and ↵ together to accept the compound formula

⌨ **Press** [Tab] to move to E3

⌨ **Edit** the formula by replacing "$F" with "$G".

The corrected formula should read:

=SUM(IF('Data Analysis'!$G$2:'Data Analysis'!$G$734=$B3, IF('Data Analysis' !$H$2:'Data Analysis'!$H$734="No",1,0),0))

⌨ **Press** [Ctrl] and [Shift] and ↵ together to accept the compound formula

⌨ **Press** [Tab] to move to F3

⌨ **Edit** the formula by replacing 'No' with 'Yes'.

The corrected formula should read:

=SUM(IF('Data Analysis'!$G$2:'Data Analysis'!$G$734=$B3, IF('Data Analysis' !$H$2:'Data Analysis'!$H$734="Yes",1,0),0))

⌨ **Press** [Ctrl] and [Shift] and ↵ together to accept the compound formula

🖑 **Highlight** D3 to F3

🖑 **AutoFill** the formula down to row 7.

The finished table looks like the one below:

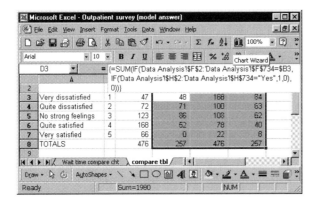

Now we will produce a chart from this data.

We will plot waiting area and waiting time separately. Waiting area first:

🖰 **Highlight** C2 to D7

⌨ **Hold down** the [Ctrl] Key, *and*

🖰 **Highlight** A2 to A7.

This multiple selection will ensure that Excel uses the correct labels for the categories.

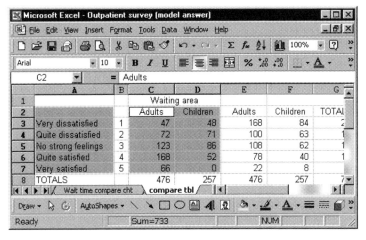

🖰 **Click** on 📊 to start the Chart Wizard.

🖰 **Click** on the 3-D column chart option as below.

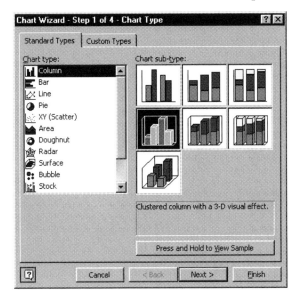

🖑 **Click** on Next >.

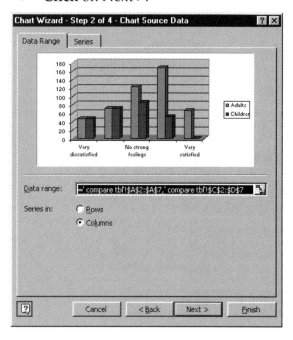

🖑 **Click** on Next >.

Enter the titles as shown:

⌨ **Type** Comparison of satisfaction with the waiting area

⌨ **Press** [tab]

⌨ **Type** Satisfaction

⌨ **Press** [tab].

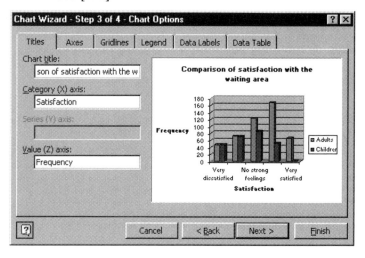

🖑 **Click** on Next >

🖑 **Click** on As new sheet.

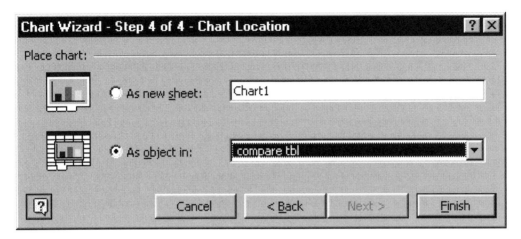

🖑 **Click** on Finish.

To tidy up, change the orientation of the vertical axis label:

🖑 **Right-click** on the frequency axis

🖑 **Click** on Format Axis Title

🖑 **Click** on Alignment.

Rotate the text through 90°.

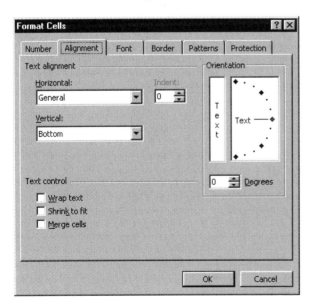

Click on [OK].

The finished graph is shown below.

Now tidy up the sheet labels by renaming Sheet4 as 'Compare tbl' and Chart1 as 'Wait area compare cht'.

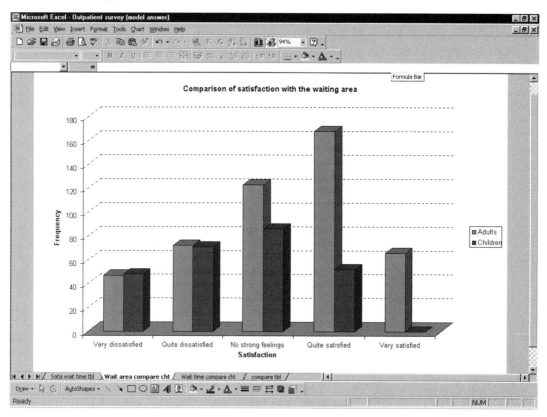

Exercise

The chart of the comparative data for the waiting time is identical in almost every detail. Enter the chart in the book as 'wait time compare cht'. A model answer for the chart is given opposite.

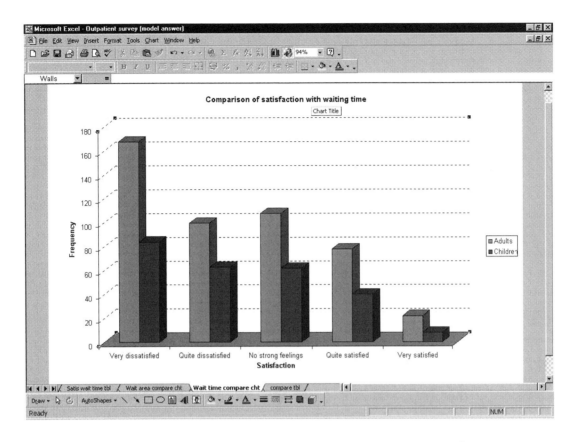

The final stage is to look for significant associations between the satisfaction ratings and carry out a chi-squared test to look for any association between the age of the patient and their satisfaction level.

The chi-squared test is used to establish whether there is a relationship between two factors. We will use it to establish whether there is a link between the satisfaction ratings for waiting time and the waiting area.

In order to carry out a chi-squared test we must define three things:

1   A table of actual values
2   A null hypothesis
3   A table of expected values for the null hypothesis.

The table of actual values is constructed by cross-tabulating the two variables in this case, the satisfaction with the waiting area or time and the age of the patient:

satisfaction	Adult	Children	Total
1			
2			A
3			
4			
5			
Total		B	C

In the table above, 1 is very satisfied, 2 is quite satisfied, 3 is no strong feelings, 4 is quite dissatisfied and 5 is very dissatisfied. A is the total number of responses quite satisfied with the waiting area (or time), B is the total number of child patients and C is the total number of patients.

Thus, the shaded cell contains the number of child patients who were quite satisfied.

The null hypothesis states that there is no relationship between the factors. If this was true then we would expect the adult and child columns to be in the same proportion.

In the chi-squared test, we measure the p-value. The p-value is the probability of observing the given data when the null hypothesis is true.

A p-value of close to zero implies that the probability of observing this data when the null hypothesis is true is very low. Generally, by convention, less than 5% is taken as significant.

We now calculate the table of values which we would expect if there was no relationship, that is, the null hypothesis is true. These values are calculated as follows:

$$\frac{\text{Row total x Column total}}{\text{Sample total}}$$

For example, in terms of the table above, the value in the shaded cell of the table of expected values is given by:

$$\frac{(A \times B)}{C}$$

In terms of Excel, we do three steps:

1 Add totals to our table of actual values
2 Use these to construct a table of expected values
3 Use the CHITEST() function to calculate the p-value or probability that the null hypothesis is true.

To add totals to our table:

🖰 **Highlight** cells E3 to E5

🖰 **Click** on Insert in the menu bar

🖰 **Click** on Shift cells right

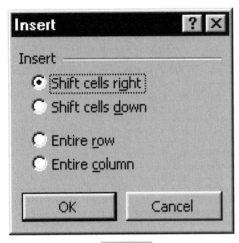

🖰 **Click** on OK

🖰 **Click** on E2

⌨ **Type** TOTALS

⌨ **Press** ↵

🖰 **Click** on Σ on the tool bar whilst in cell E3

⌨ Change the formula to read =SUM(C3:D3)

🖰 **AutoFill** the formula down to E7

🖰 **Click** on H2

⌨ **Type** TOTALS

⌨ **Press** ↵

🖰 Click on Σ on the tool bar whilst in cell H3

⌨ **Press** ↵

🖰 **AutoFill** the formula down to H7

🖰 **Click** on A8

⌨ **Type** TOTALS

⌨ **Press** [Tab] twice

🖰 **Click** on Σ on the tool bar whilst in cell C8

⌨ **Press** ↵

🖰 **Click** on C8

🖰 **AutoFill** the formula across to H8.

Now we can construct our table of expected values:

🖰 **Click** on C10

⌨ **Type** =$E3*C$8/$E$8   (row total x column total/overall total)

⌨ **Press** ↵

🖰 **Click** on C10

🖰 **AutoFill** the formula across to D10

🖰 **AutoFill** the pair of formulae down to row 14

🖰 **Click** on F10

⌨ **Type** =$H3*F$8/$H$8   (row total x column total/overall total)

⌨ **Press** ↵

🖰 **Click** on F10

🖰 **AutoFill** the formula across to G10

🖰 **AutoFill** the pair of formulae down to row 14.

Now for the final step:

🖰 **Click** on A16

⌨ **Type** P-values

⌨ **Press** [Tab] twice

🖰 **Click** on *fx*

🖰 **Click** on Statistical in the Function category list if the CHITEST function is not visible in the Most Recently Used category

🖰 **Click** on the scroll bar bottom arrow until CHITEST is visible

🖰 **Click** on CHITEST

🖰 **Click** on ⬚ OK ⬚

⌨ **Type** C3:D7

⌨ **Press** [Tab]

⌨ **Type** C10:D14

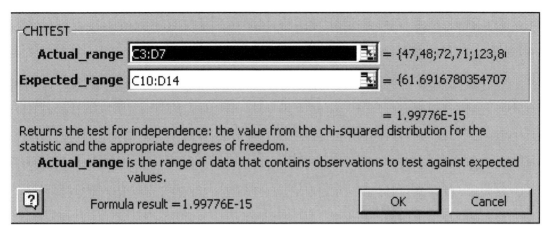

⌨ **Press ⏎.**

This gives a value of 2×10^{-15}. This indicates an association between satisfaction with the waiting area and the patient's age.

For the waiting time data:

🖰 **Click** on F16

🖰 **Click** on f_*

🖰 **Click** on CHITEST

🖰 **Click** on [OK]

⌨ **Type** F3:G7

⌨ **Press** [Tab]

⌨ **Type** F10:G14

⌨ **Press ⏎.**

This time the answer is 0.66, not indicative of an association. This means that the results obtained do not depart significantly from those expected from simple proportions.

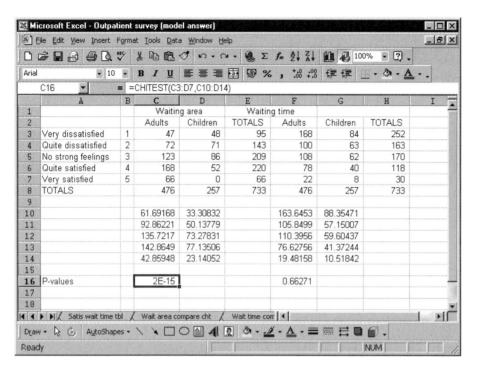

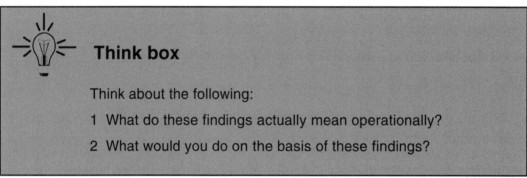

Think box

Think about the following:

1 What do these findings actually mean operationally?

2 What would you do on the basis of these findings?

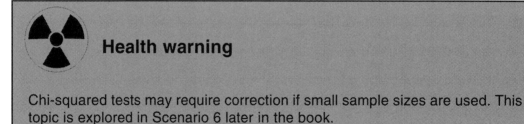

Health warning

Chi-squared tests may require correction if small sample sizes are used. This topic is explored in Scenario 6 later in the book.

Weighing the evidence

In this chapter

This chapter will tell you how to:

*   look at statistics from published studies

*   check existing statistics in existing studies

*   use Excel to evaluate the validity and significance of existing studies

*   use statistics in your own studies

 plot scatter graphs to look at comparisons of continuous data

 carry out correlation and regression analysis in Excel

 carry out t-tests in Excel

 calculate confidence intervals and sample sizes.

The scenario

You have been elected by your colleagues to compile evidence-based guide-lines to provide a basis for clinical governance. You have decided to review a sample of small clinical research projects to look at whether they can suitably form the basis of good clinical practice. You wish to locally validate the studies by using Excel to reproduce the statistical analyses and to test the statistical power of the studies.

In a review of four volumes of the *New England Journal of Medicine*[1] it was found that 12% of all studies used correlation analysis to investigate the relationship between two variables, and that 8% of all studies used linear regression techniques. This therefore seems like a good point to start.

Correlation analysis is used to analyse the association between two or more variables. One type of correlation co-efficient, implemented within Excel, is the Pearson co-efficient. We will consider its use in a study by Mazess *et al.*[2] The study investigated the association between a patient's age and the percentage of their body weight stored as fat. It might be expected that as age increases, so does the percentage of body weight stored as fat. The data from the study is shown in the table below. The first job is to enter the data into a new Excel spreadsheet:

Mazess et al., 1984		
Subject	Age	%Fat
1	23	9.5
2	23	27.9
3	27	7.8
4	27	17.8
5	39	31.4
6	41	25.9
7	45	27.4
8	49	25.2
9	50	31.1
10	53	34.7
11	53	42
12	54	29.1
13	56	32.5
14	57	30.3
15	58	33
16	58	33.8
17	60	41.1
18	61	34.5

- **Click** on ▭ on the toolbar
- **Click** on A1
- **Type** Subject
- **Press** [tab]
- **Type** Age
- **Press** [tab]
- **Type** %Fat
- **Press** [tab]
- **Click** on A2
- **Type** 1
- **Press** [tab]
- **Type** 23
- **Press** [tab]
- **Type** 9.5
- **Press** [tab]

[1] Emerson JA and Colditz GA (1993) Use of statistical analysis in the New England Journal of Medicine. *N Eng J Med.* **309**: 709–13.
[2] Mazess RB, Peppler WW and Gibbons M (1984)Total body composition by dual-photon (153Gd) absorptiometry. *Am J Clin Nut.* **40**: 834–9.

And so on until it looks like the one I prepared earlier:

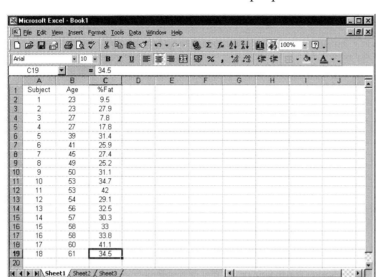

The first task is to look at a graph of the data to visually analyse the data.
   The graph we will use is a two-dimensional scatter plot. To plot the data:

🖱 **Highlight** B1 to C19

🖱 **Click** on 📊 to start the Chart Wizard

🖱 **Click** on XY (Scatter) in the list of <u>C</u>hart types

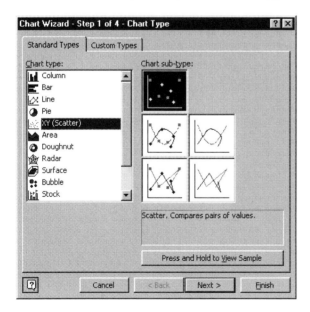

🖰 **Click** on Next >

🖰 **Click** on Next > again to accept the Chart Source Data options.

At the Chart Options step:

⌨ Edit the titles so that they are as shown in the screen shot below

🖰 **Click** on the Legend tab

🖰 **Click** in the Show legend box to remove the legend

🖰 **Click** on Next >

🖰 **Click** the As new sheet option

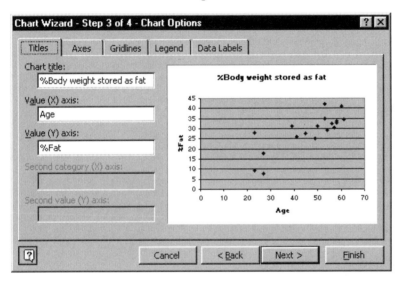

🖰 **Click** on Finish.

For this type of chart we may want to change the background and gridlines:

🖰 **Right-click** within the chart area

🖰 **Click** on Format Plot Area

🖰 **Click** on None in the Border box

🖰 **Click** on None in the Area box

🖰 **Click** on OK .

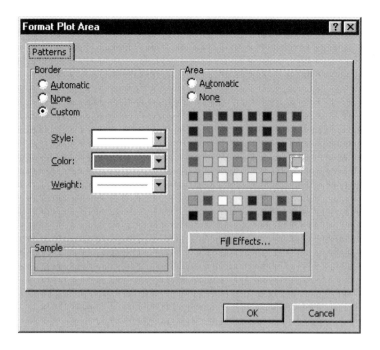

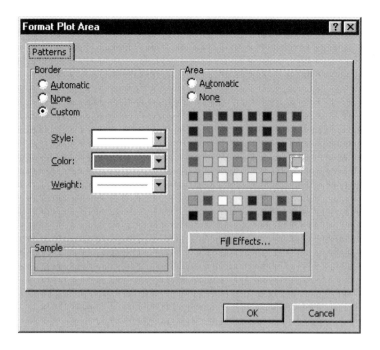 **Right-click** on one of the gridlines

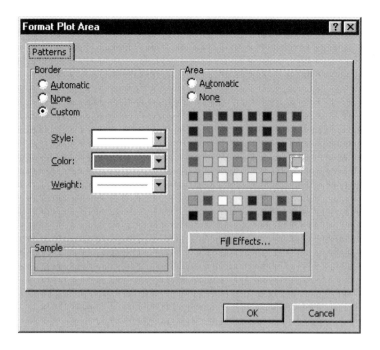 **Click** on Format Gridlines

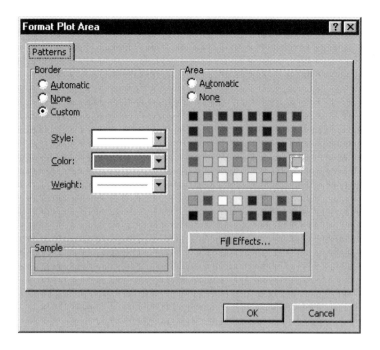 **Click** on the custom box

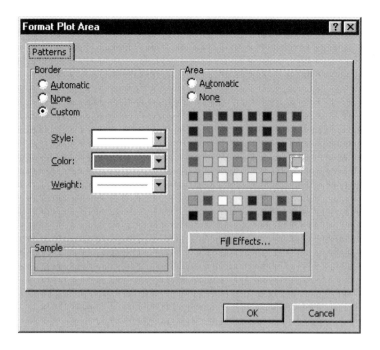 **Click** on ▼ in the Style box

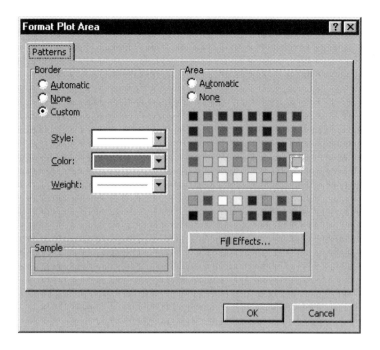 **Click** on – – – – – in the resulting list

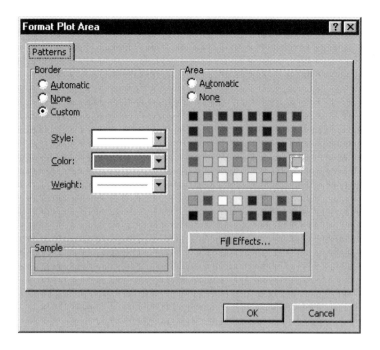 **Click** on the Scale tab

 Click on the tick next to Maximum

 Press [tab]

 Type 50

 Click on the tick next to Major unit

 Press [tab]

 Type 10

 Click on OK .

To add vertical gridlines:

- ☝ **Click** on <u>C</u>hart in the menu bar
- ☝ **Click** on Chart <u>O</u>ptions in the Chart menu
- ☝ **Click** on Gridlines
- ☝ **Click** in the <u>M</u>ajor gridlines box in the Value (X) axis
- ☝ **Click** on ⬚ OK .

To make the x-axis gridlines dotted:

- ☝ **Right-click** on one of the x-axis gridlines
- ☝ **Click** on Fo<u>r</u>mat Gridlines
- ☝ **Click** on the custom box
- ☝ **Click** on ▾ in the Style box
- ☝ **Click** on – – – – – in the resulting list
- ☝ **Click** on ⬚ OK .

The result should look like the one below.

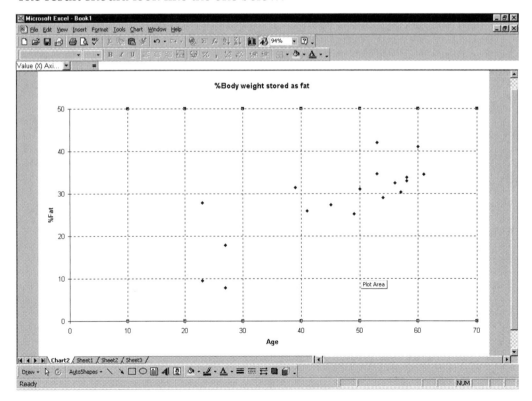

> ## Hint
>
>
>
> The appearance of the scatter plot tells us a lot about any correlation.
>
> If the data clusters around a line going from bottom left to top right, there is a positive correlation.
>
> If the data clusters around a line going from top left to bottom right, there is a negative correlation.
>
> If the data is scattered all over, then there is no correlation.

As the graph shows, there is some degree of association between the two variables but that it is not very strong. We can now measure the strength of that association by using the Pearson correlation coefficient:

Correlations and scatter plots according to goldfish!

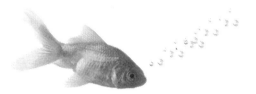

Positive correlation

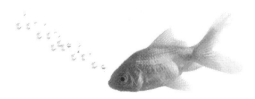

Negative correlation

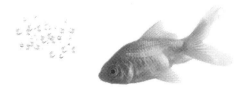

No obvious correlation

🖑 **Click** on E2

⌨ **Type**   r=   (*r denotes correlation co-efficient*)

🖑 **Click** on F2.

🖑 **Click** on *fx*

🖑 **Click** on Statistical in the Function c̲ategory

🖑 **Click** on CORREL in the list of Function n̲ames

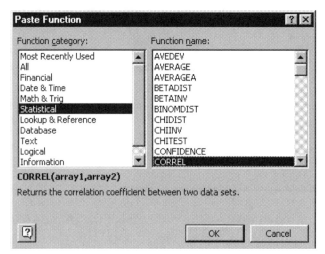

🖑 **Click** on   OK

⌨ **Type** B2:B19

⌨ **Press** [tab]

⌨ **Type** C2:C19

🖑 **Click** on   OK .

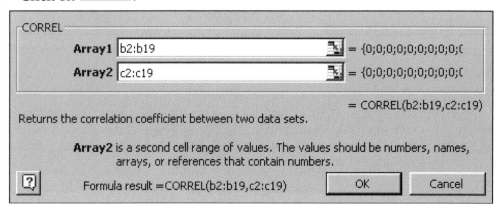

The correct answer is 0.792086.

Principle of good practice

This has far too many decimal places. Use to reduce it to a sensible 0.79.

Hint

The value of the correlation coefficient varies between -1 and +1 where 0 indicates no statistical association, +1 indicates a strong positive association and -1 indicates a strong negative association. In this case we have a strong(ish) association.

Values of closer to zero than ± 0.7 are generally not worth investigating.

However, this example does also illustrate one of the pitfalls of this kind of analysis. The patient group was a mixed sex group. The gender of the patient is a potential confounding factor.

Exercise

An alternative method is to use the Analysis Toolpak. This uses a similar method to our earlier example based on descriptive statistics. This is left as an exercise. The method may be found on the website. The answer is the same.

Hint

This approach to correlation using the Data Analysis option is most useful when there are a number of variables to be examined. A matrix is created showing correlations between all variables.

The male patients are shown as M and the females as F. To investigate the effect of the patient's sex, we must first sort our patients according to sex:

🖑 **Highlight** A1:D19

🖑 **Click** on Data in the menu bar

🖑 **Click** on Sort

🖑 **Click** on ▼ next to Subject in the 'Sort By' box.

From the list that appears:

🖑 **Click** on Sex

🖑 **Click** on ⬚ OK ⬚ .

Now we can easily find the correlation co-efficient for male and female patients:

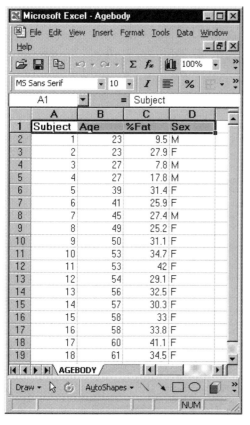

🖑 **Click** on E4

⌨ Edit the cell so that it reads r(F)=

🖑 **Click** on F4

⌨ Edit the formula to read =CORREL (B2:B15,C2:C15)

🖑 **Click** on E5

⌨ Edit the cell so that it reads r(M)=

🖑 **Click** on E4

⌨ Edit the formula to read =CORREL (B16:B19,C2:C19).

The completed sheet is shown opposite.

The correlation co-efficient for female patients is now 0.51, much lower than for the whole sample. The male figure derived from only four patients is 0.89. (A figure derived from only four patients is inherently spurious, being too small a sample to be significantly different from 0).

Men have a lower percentage of their body weight as fat than women. Because the men in this sample happened to be younger, the mixed sample appeared more strongly linked than is the case. Thus, the small and skewed sample gave a spurious credibility to the relationship. A larger sample will tend to randomise other factors and therefore produce a more reliable result.

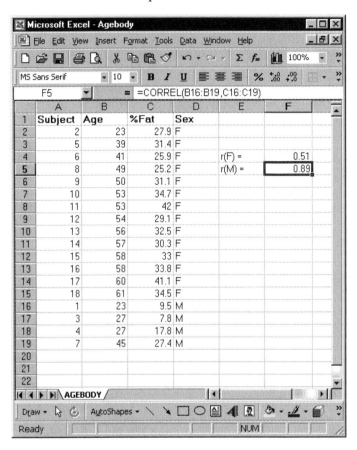

Regression

In formal terms, regression analysis is used to describe the relationship between one dependent variable and one or more predictive (or independent) variables, and assess by how much the value of a dependent variable will change in response to changes in the predictive variables.

In Excel there are two methods by which we can do this – one of which produces limited results and the other which produces comprehensive results, and can be used to tell us more about the data.

Hint

In simple terms, regression is used to put a line of best fit through the data.

For convenience, we will continue with our example study, but consider only the female data, although in other circumstances we would not bother to pursue a correlation with a co-efficient of 0.59.

The LINEST function from the Function Wizard gives us the gradient of the line of best fit, known as m. The equation of the line is given by Y= mX + c, where m is the gradient and c the intercept with the y-axis:

🖱 **Click** on E7

⌨ **Type** m=

⌨ **Press** [tab]

🖱 **Click** on on f_x

🖱 **Click** on Statistical in the list of categories

🖱 **Click** on LINEST in the list of statistical functions

🖱 **Click** on ⌧ OK ⌧.

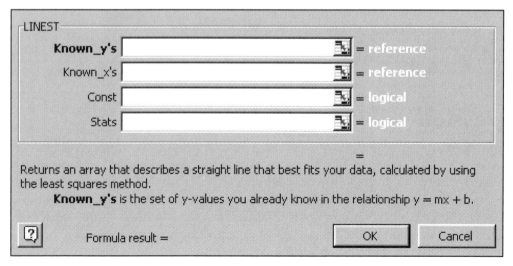

⌨ **Type** B2:B15

⌨ **Press** [tab]

⌨ **Type** C2:C15

⌨ **Press** ↵.

To calculate the intercept:

⌨ **Press** [⇧] and [tab] to move to E8

⌨ **Type** m=

⌨ **Press** [tab]

🖱 **Click** on *fx*

🖱 **Click** on Statistical in the list of categories

🖱 **Click** on INTERCEPT in the list of statistical functions

🖱 **Click** on ⬚ OK ⬚

⌨ **Type** B2:B15

⌨ **Press** [tab]

⌨ **Type** C2:C15

⌨ **Press** ↵.

The final results are:

m = 0.24

c = 20.11

producing a regression line of

y= 0.24 x + 20.11

The resulting sheet is shown below:

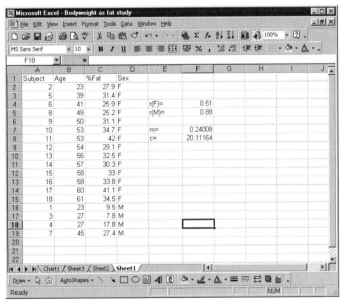

The problem is that we don't know how good a fit the line is. This is crucial to the quality of any evidence produced as a result of a study like this.

To investigate this we will use an alternative approach, based on the Analysis Toolpak:

🖱 **Click** on Tools in the menu bar

🖱 **Click** on Data Analysis in the Tools menu

🖱 **Click** on Regression in the list of tools available

🖱 **Click** on ⬛ OK ⬛

⌨ **Type** C2:C15 in the Input Y Range box

⌨ **Type** B2:B15 in the Input X Range box.

The box should look like the one below:

🖱 **Click** on ⬛ OK ⬛.

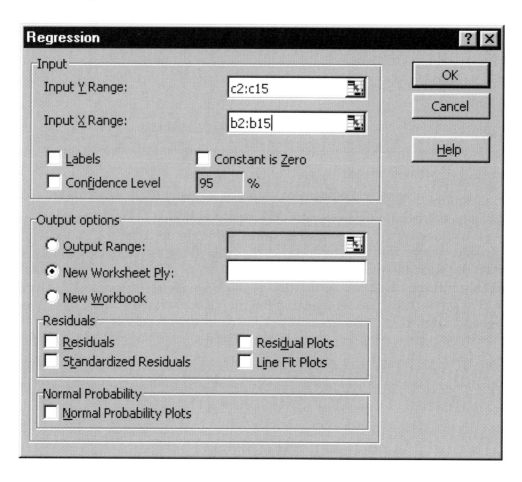

The results are produced in Sheet2.

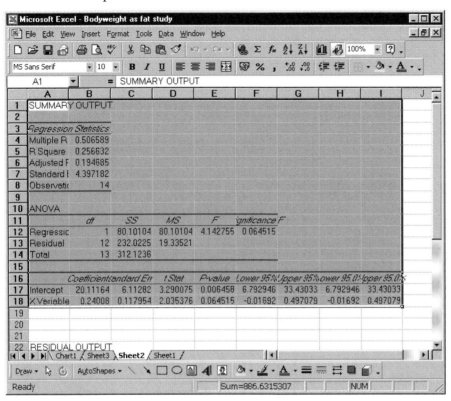

This option produces useful data not just about the line itself but the strength of the association.

Crucially, the p-value from the ANOVA analysis shown in cell F12 in the significance P column is 0.064 (6.4%). This value being greater than 5%, indicates that you should accept the null hypothesis, i.e. that there is no linear relationship between the variables.

This is confirmed by the fact that the p-value for the co-efficient of x, given in cell E18, is 0.064 (6.4). This tells us that the line *could* be flat; in which case, y does not depend upon x.

Looking for evidence of an association amongst continuous data

One of the other common types occurs when an intervention is made. Data is collected before and after, and then compared to see whether the impact of the intervention has been significant.

We will use an example from the *British Medical Journal* to illustrate how a paired t-test can be used to evaluate such an intervention.

 Health warning

The paired t-test is only one type of t-test. However, it is a common type since paired data arises from many interventions where data is measured before and after.

It is also the easiest to implement in Excel, although other techniques are available.

If this opportunistic approach does not meet your needs, you may want to consult that passing statistician again and perhaps invest in a specialist package.

The case to be investigated is a study of the administration of a growth hormone.[3] In this study, heights of 16 children were measured before administration, and one year later. The results were standardised for age.

The following results, as shown in the table on page 161, were found.

We will open a new workbook to enter our data:

🖱 **Click** on ▯ on the toolbar

🖱 **Double-click** on the tab labelled Sheet1 at the bottom of the sheet

⌨ **Type** Data

---

[3] Hindmarsh PC and Brook CGD (1987) Effect of human growth hormone on short normal children. *British Medical Journal.* **295:** 573–7.

Subject	Baseline	At 1 year		
1	-0.7	4.1	🖰	**Click** on A1
2	0.0	3.4	⌨	**Type** Subject
3	-0.7	3.1	⌨	**Press** [tab]
4	-0.7	3.0	⌨	**Type** Baseline
5	0.5	2.8	⌨	**Press** [tab]
6	-0.7	2.7	⌨	**Type** After 1 year
7	-0.6	2.5	⌨	**Press** ↵
8	-0.3	2.3	🖰	**Click** on A2
9	-0.7	2.2	⌨	**Type** 1
10	-0.7	2.0	⌨	**Press** ↵
11	-0.5	1.8	🖰	**Type** =A2+1
12	-0.7	1.6	⌨	**Press** ↵
13	-0.5	1.3	🖰	**Click** on A3
14	-0.7	0.9	🖰	**AutoFill** down to A17
15	-0.4	0.8	🖰	**Click** on B2
16	-0.3	0.3	⌨	**Type** 0.7
			⌨	**Press** ↵ to move to B3.

And so on ... Complete the table so that your sheet looks like the one I prepared earlier, shown below:

🖰 **Click** on File in the menu bar

🖰 **Click** on Save As on the File menu.

In the Save As dialog box:

⌨ **Type** Growth Hormone and **Press** ↵.

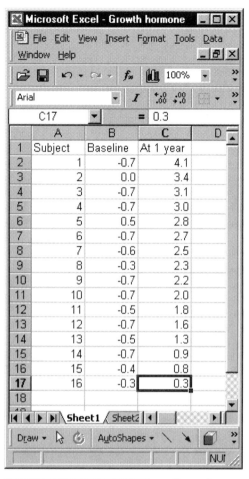

First, we calculate the difference for each subject:

🖰 **Click** on D1

✎ **Type** Difference

✎ **Press** ↵

✎ **Type** =C2-B2

✎ **Press** ↵

🖰 **Click** on D2 again

🖰 **AutoFill** down to A17.

The completed sheet looks like the one below.

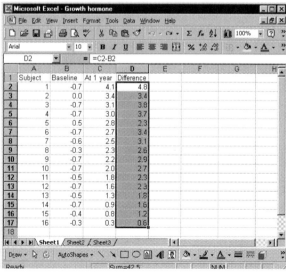

Health warning

The paired t-test to be used can only be applied when the differences to be investigated show a normal distribution.

This may be identified by a distribution where the mean, median and mode are similar and the skew is near to zero.

This may be investigated in Excel using the descriptive statistics found on the data analysis option of the Tools menu.

First, we will confirm that the differences produce a normal distribution:

Exercise

The first step is to investigate whether the differences show a normal distribution, using the Data Analysis option on the Tools menu.

Put the solution in a separate sheet and rename it analysis.

This has been done previously, so is left as an exercise, with the main dialog box and the solution shown in the Hint box below.

Hint

The main dialog box should look like:

The finished sheet should look like this:

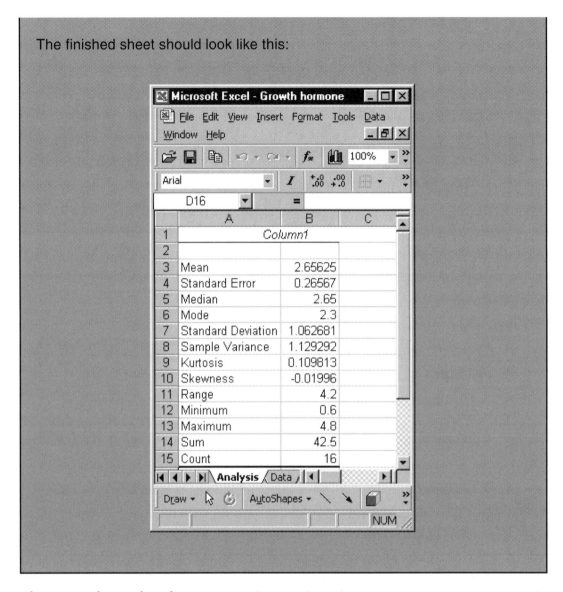

The result shows that the mean, median and mode are 2.66. 2.65, 2.3 respectively and the skew is a low -0.02. As always, the figures should be interpreted in the light of common sense, i.e. do we expect it to be a normal distribution?

Therefore, we can proceed to carry out our t-test:

- 🖰 **Click** on the <u>D</u>ata tab to return to the data sheet
- 🖰 **Click** on <u>T</u>ools in the menu bar
- 🖰 **Click** on <u>D</u>ata Analysis in the <u>T</u>ools menu
- 🖰 **Click** on t-Test: paired Two sample for Means in the list of tools.

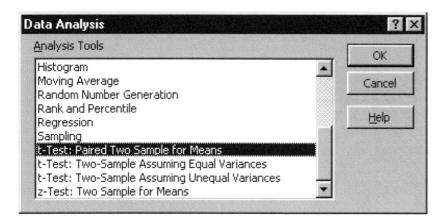

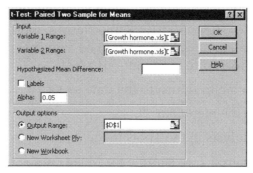 **Click** on [OK].

At the Variable 1 Range box:

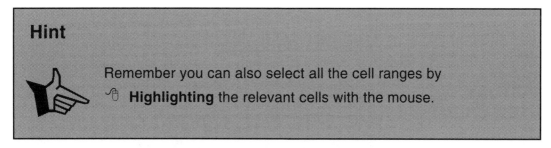 **Type** B2:B17

 Press [tab]

 Type C2:C17 in the Variable 2 Range box

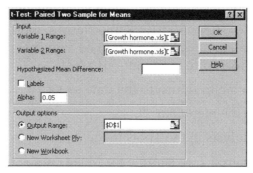 **Click** in the Output Range box

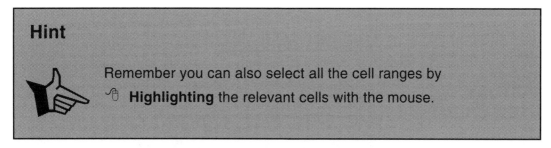 **Type** Analysis!B2:B17.

Hint

Remember you can also select all the cell ranges by
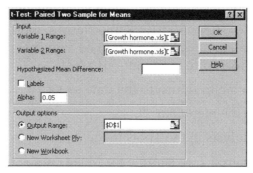 **Highlighting** the relevant cells with the mouse.

The completed box should look like this:

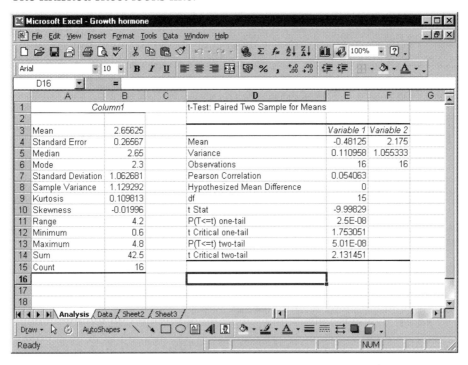 **Click** on [OK].

The finished sheet looks like:

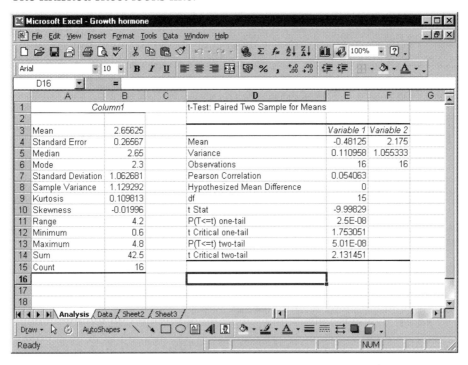

By convention, a p-value of less than 0.05 is regarded as significant. In this case, a two-tailed test, this is easily achieved.

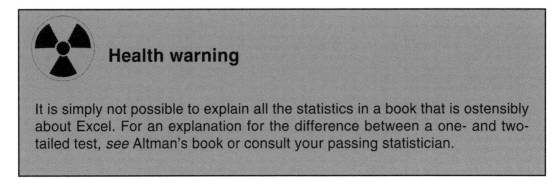

Health warning

It is simply not possible to explain all the statistics in a book that is ostensibly about Excel. For an explanation for the difference between a one- and two-tailed test, *see* Altman's book or consult your passing statistician.

Sample size

If we want to move from assessing other people's research size to designing our own research, then one of the first questions we need to ask is how big a sample size do we need to investigate?

We will consider the case of the classical random control trial (RCT) and build a little calculator in Excel to work out how big our sample size needs to be to give a significant result.

The sample size depends upon the type of RCT undertaken. In the following case, we count the proportion of people responding from two identically-sized groups. If your RCT is based upon a different design, you will need to tweak the calculator for your own needs.

We will build our calculator in three steps:

1   build a basic sheet
2   explain how it works
3   pretty it up to look like the one I prepared earlier.

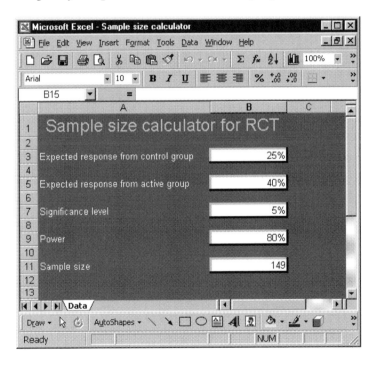

First, we need a basic sheet. We'll open a new sheet and add some labels:

🖱 **Click** on ⬜ on the toolbar

🖱 **Double-click** on the tab labelled Sheet1 at the bottom of the sheet

⌨ **Type** Data

🖱 **Click** on A1

⌨ **Type** Sample size calculator for RCT

⌨ **Press** ↵ twice

⌨ **Type** Expected response from control group

⌨ **Press** ↵ twice

⌨ **Type** Expected response from active group

⌨ **Press** ↵ twice

⌨ **Type** Significance level

⌨ **Press** ↵ twice

⌨ **Type** Power

⌨ **Press** ↵ twice

⌨ **Type** Sample size

⌨ **Press** ↵

🖱 **Click** on B3

⌨ **Type** 25%

⌨ **Press** ↵ twice

⌨ **Type** 50%

⌨ **Press** ↵ twice

⌨ **Type** 5%

⌨ **Press** ↵ twice

⌨ **Type** 80%

⌨ **Press** ↵.

By now, the screen should look something like the one on the right.

Next we do some calculations using Excel functions:

🖑 **Click** on C3

⌨ **Type** z-alpha

⌨ **Press** ↵ twice

⌨ **Type** z-2beta

⌨ **Press** ↵ twice

⌨ **Type** z term

⌨ **Press** ↵ twice

⌨ **Type** delta

🖑 **Press** ↵

🖑 **Click** on D3

⌨ **Type** =ABS(NORMSINV(B7/2))

⌨ **Press** ↵ twice

⌨ **Type** =1-B9

⌨ **Press** ↵ twice

⌨ **Type** =ABS(NORMSINV(D5))

⌨ **Press** ↵ twice

⌨ **Type** =(D3+D7)*(D3+D7)

⌨ Press ↵ twice

⌨ Type =B5-B3

To calculate the sample size itself:

🖑 **Click** on B11

⌨ **Type** =D9*((B3*(1-B3))+(B5*(1-B5)))/(D11*D11)

⌨ **Press** ↵.

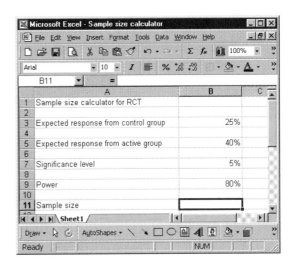

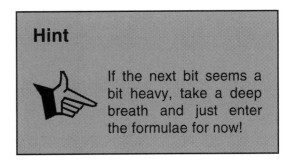

Hint

If the next bit seems a bit heavy, take a deep breath and just enter the formulae for now!

By now, the sheet should look like this:

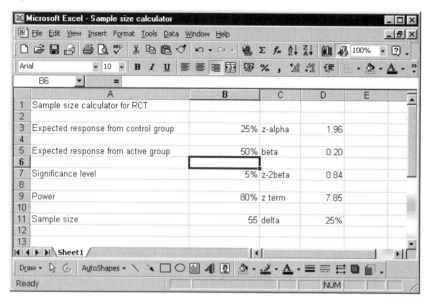

The calculator tells us that for this study we need 55 patients.

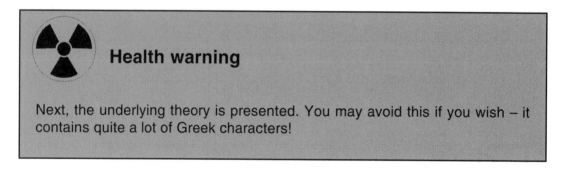

Health warning

Next, the underlying theory is presented. You may avoid this if you wish – it contains quite a lot of Greek characters!

Hint

The calculation is based on four parameters:

- expected response from control group
- expected response from active group
- significance level
- power.

The expected response from the control group is denoted by π_1. It is the expected positive results from the control group.

The expected response from the active group is denoted by π_2. It is the expected positive results from the group who experienced the intervention. The difference $\pi_1 - \pi_2$ is denoted by δ.

The significance is denoted by α. This is the level at which a significant result is deemed to have occurred, typically p-values less than 5%, or 0.05.

The power of a study is equal to $1 - \beta$. β is defined as the probability of avoiding a Type II error, that is the probability of not rejecting the null hypothesis when it is in fact false. In the absence of specific information, the power is often assumed to be 80%, corresponding to a value for β of 20%.

The sample size is given by the following expression:

$$M = (z_\alpha + z_{2\beta})^2 \, [\pi_1 \, (1 - \pi_1) + \pi_2 \, (1 - \pi_2)]/\delta^2$$

Where the z-values are the inverse normal probability functions. In our sheet,

- α is entered into B7. β is calculated in D5
- z_α and $z_{2\beta}$ are calculated in D3 and D7 respectively
- π_1 and π_2 are entered into B3 and B5 respectively
- δ is calculated in D11.

Exercise

Now to finish off our calculator with some fancy formatting. This is left as an exercise with some broad hints.

The steps required are:
1 select the whole sheet
2 format the background to teal
3 highlight Columns C and D
4 set text colour to teal to render interim figures invisible
5 change the background of cells B3, B5, B7, B9, B11 to white
6 change the boundaries of cells B3, B5, B7, B9, B11 to grey lines for the top and left, and black for the right and bottom to create the desired 3-D effect
7 emphasise the title by increasing font size and centring across Columns A and B.

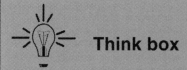 For further help see the website. Here you will find a more comprehensive calculator with pages to calculate sample sizes for other types of trial.

Think box

Your finished calculator should look like the one below. Try changing α, β, π_1, and π_2 to investigate the effect on the sample size.

Explain your findings.

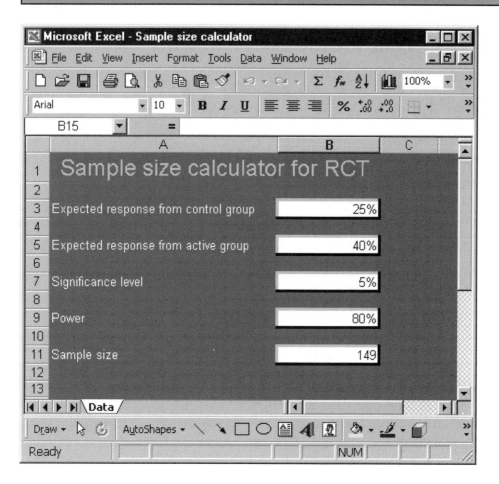

Comparison with national performance

In this chapter

This chapter will tell you how to:

- access external data sources

- compile Excel sheets from external data sources

- compare your performace with national data

- work out where you are relative to other bodies

 import worksheets from other formats into an Excel workbook

 review use of Excel functions to produce comparative benchmarks

 use hidden columns to assign a rank order.

WWW In this chapter we will also show you how to download data from the Internet.

The scenario

Much of the data collected by the NHS are made available by the NHS Executive on their website. This allows individual NHS organisations to compare their performance with their peers.

The first step is to get onto the Internet. We shall assume that you have a PC equipped to gain Internet access. This means that you have a PC equipped with a modem, and a connection to the Internet via NHSNet, a commercial Internet service provider such as Freeserve, or perhaps a local university, college, library or cybercafe.

In this scenario, you have been asked to provide a presentation to Trust management showing the relative performance of your Trust, My Own NHS Trust against national performance data.

Finding the national data

Hint

 If you don't have access to the Internet, don't despair. Simply skip the next few sections and rejoin the text at *Assembling the workbook.*

To access the Internet, click on your browser, which will be identified by the following symbol:

 Click on

Hopefully, this will take you through a process to get you onto the Internet. This may be automatic or you may be asked for a password. The modem will make a whole series of funny noises. This is all quite normal.

Hint

Your browser icon may look different. For example, it may be a proprietary symbol such as the Freeserve icon.

Alternatively, you can use a different browser such as an earlier version of Internet Explorer or Netscape Navigator:

In this chapter, all screens are based upon using Internet Explorer 5.

You will first arrive at your home page. Mine looks like this:

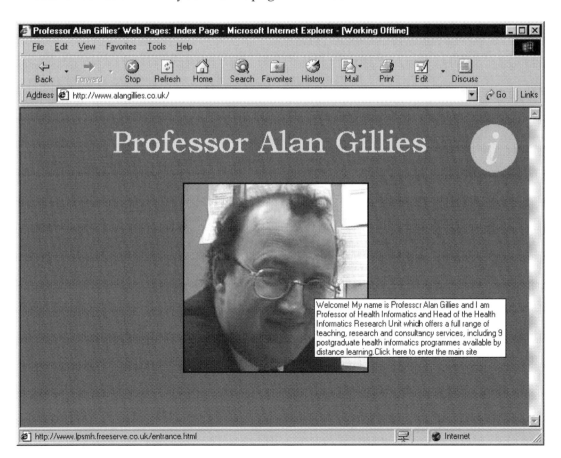

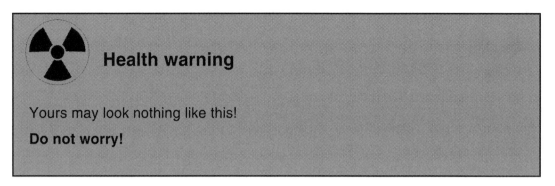

Health warning

Yours may look nothing like this!

Do not worry!

🖱 **Click** in the Address box:

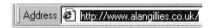

⌨ **Type** www.doh.gov.uk/tables98/index.htm

⌨ **Press** ↵.

The following page should appear:

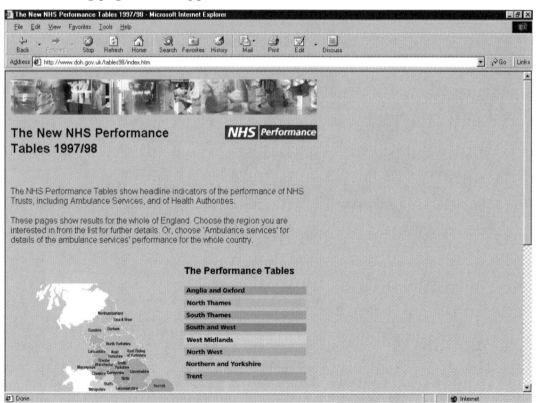

Health warning

The Internet is dynamic. If the page does not appear, look at the web pages for this book to find information on an updated link, or contact the author by email to complain!

Click on the right-hand scroll bar bottom button (⯆) to scroll down through the page to the bottom.

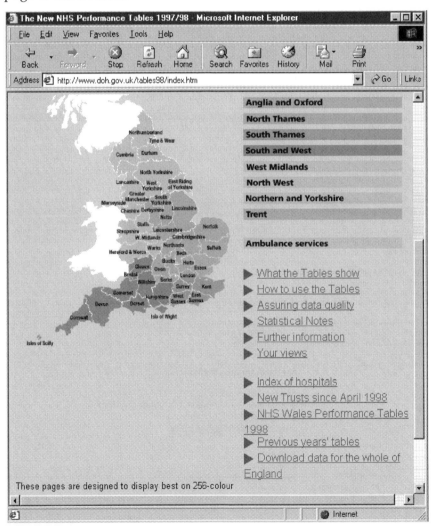

🖰 **Click** on Download data for the whole of England.

🖰 **Click** on the right-hand scroll bar bottom button (⬇) to scroll down through the page to the section entitled Spreadsheet version.

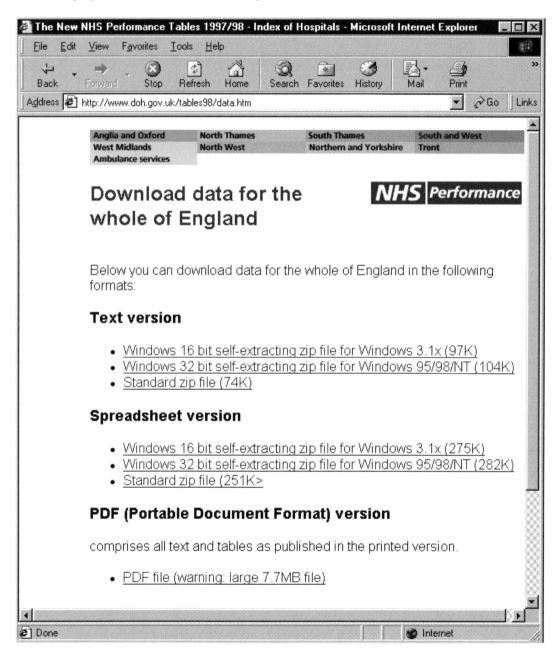

🖑 **Click** on <u>Windows 32 bit self extracting zip file for Windows 95/98/NT</u> <u>(282k)</u>.

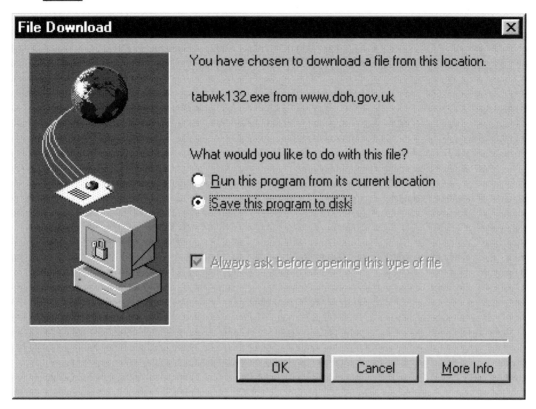

If the <u>S</u>ave this program to disk option is not selected,

🖑 **Click** on it now

🖑 **Click** on 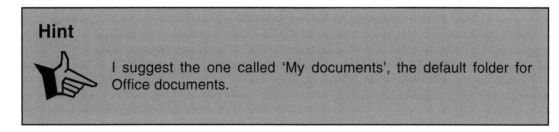 OK

🖑 **Click** on the folder of your choice to store the files.

> ## Hint
>
> I suggest the one called 'My documents', the default folder for Office documents.

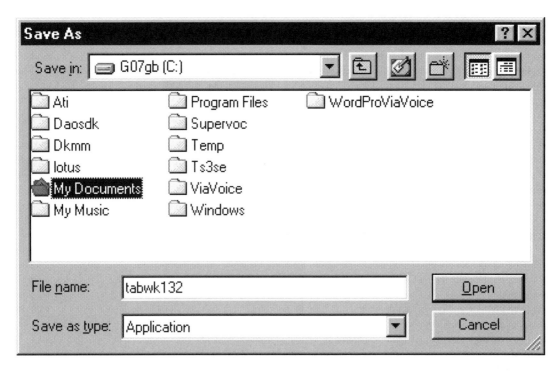

🖱 **Click** on <u>O</u>pen.

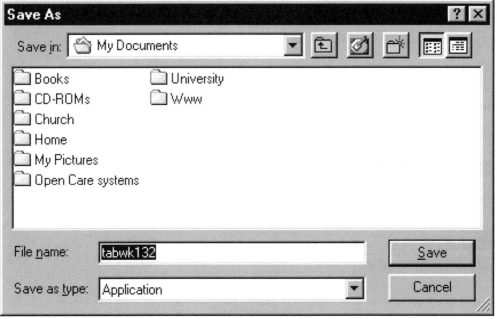

🖱 **Click** on <u>S</u>ave.

Once the transfer is complete, you can disconnect from the Internet. To prevent you incurring any more phone charges close down the data transfer window and the Internet Explorer windows:

🖱 **Click** on ☒ in the top right-hand corner of the relevant windows.

If you look in the Documents folder you will find a new file called tabwk132:

🖱 **Click** on 🖥 on the desktop

🖱 **Click** on ⌨ G07qb (C:)

🖱 **Click** on the appropriate folder, e.g. My documents.

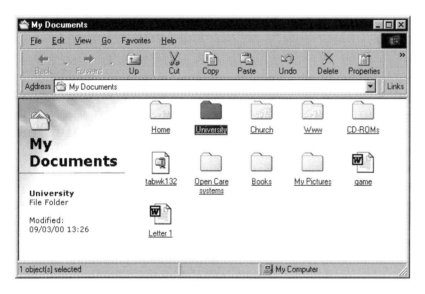

🖱 **Double-click** on the icon called tabwk132.

A dialog box appears asking for a destination folder.

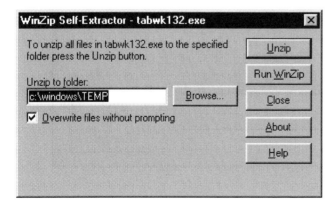

🖑 **Click** on <u>B</u>rowse

🖑 **Click** on 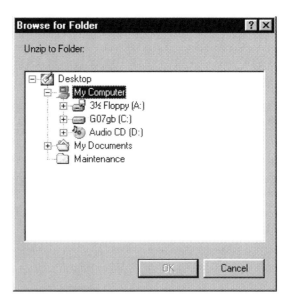 G07gb (C:)

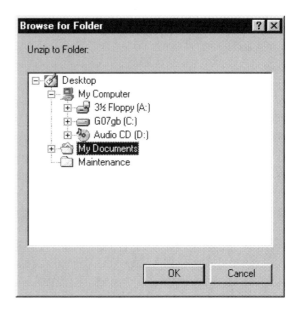

🖑 **Click** on the appropriate
folder, e.g. My documents

🖑 **Click** on [OK]

🖑 **Click** on <u>U</u>nzip

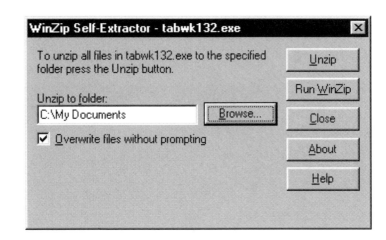

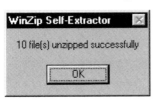

🖑 **Click** on OK

🖑 **Click** on <u>C</u>lose.

The folder where the files are stored e.g. My documents, now contains 10 new files. Each one is a Lotus 1-2-3 spreadsheet which we will use to construct one single Excel workbook.

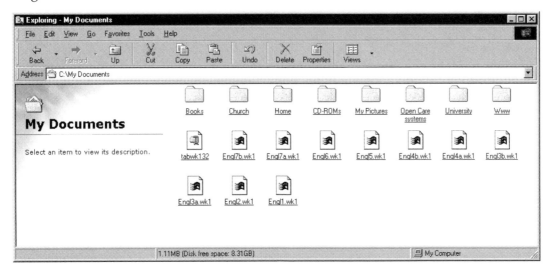

Assembling the Excel workbook

First we need to return to Excel. If Excel is not open, then:

🖑 **Double-click** on 📊 to open Excel

🖑 **Click** on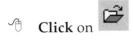

At the Open dialog box:

🖱 **Click** on ▾ at the Files of type list box

🖱 **Click** on Lotus 1-2-3 files in the resulting list.

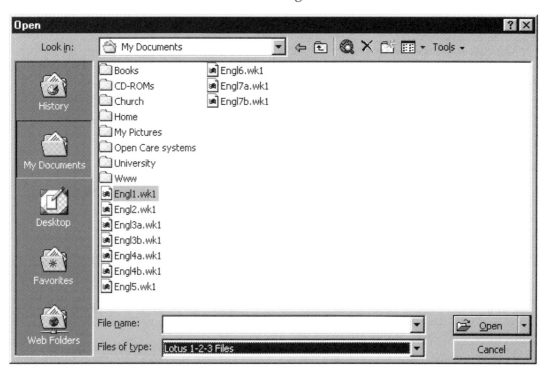

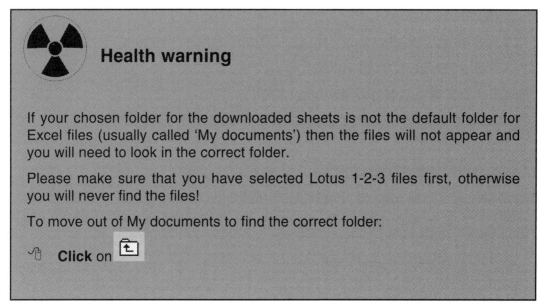

Health warning

If your chosen folder for the downloaded sheets is not the default folder for Excel files (usually called 'My documents') then the files will not appear and you will need to look in the correct folder.

Please make sure that you have selected Lotus 1-2-3 files first, otherwise you will never find the files!

To move out of My documents to find the correct folder:

🖱 **Click** on ▣

🖱 **Click** on Engl1.wk1 in the list of files

⌨ **Hold down** the [⇧] key and 🖱 **Click** on Engl7b.wk1.

This should select all the downloaded files:

🖱 **Click** on <u>O</u>pen to open all the files.

This opens each file as a separate workbook and we want to place them all as individual sheets in the same book. To do this:

🖱 **Click** on <u>E</u>dit in the menu bar

🖱 **Click** on <u>M</u>ove or Copy sheet

🖱 **Click** on ▾ in the <u>T</u>o book box

🖱 **Click** on ENGL1.WK1

🖱 **Click** on (Move to end)

🖱 **Click** on OK .

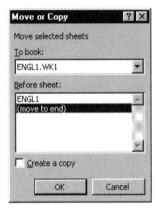

Now we move each of the other sheets into this workbook:

🖱 **Click** on <u>W</u>indow in the menu bar

🖱 **Click** on Engl7a.wk1

🖱 **Click** on Edit in the menu bar

🖱 **Click** on <u>M</u>ove or Copy sheet

🖱 **Click** on ▾ in the <u>T</u>o book box

🖱 **Click** on ENGL7B

🖱 **Click** on OK .

Now we can add sheets Engl6.wk1, Engl5.wk1, Engl4b.wk1, Engl4a.wk1, Engl3b.wk1, Engl3a.wk1 and Engl2.wk1 by the same process.

Finally, we need to save the workbook as an Excel workbook:

🖱 **Click** on <u>F</u>ile in the menu bar

🖱 **Click** on Save <u>A</u>s

⌨ **Type** National NHS Indicator dataset 1997

🖰 **Click** on ▼ in the Save as type box

🖰 **Click** on Excel 97 & 5.0/95 workbook

🖰 **Click** on ⌷ OK ⌷.

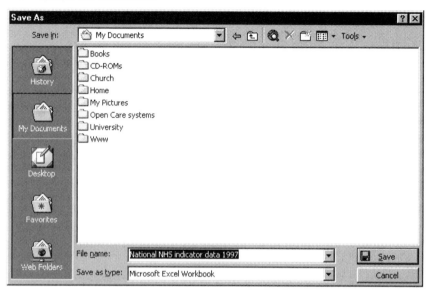

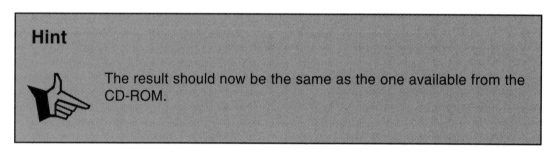

Hint

The result should now be the same as the one available from the CD-ROM.

Now we have an Excel book derived from the national data, we can use it to compare performance with those of our Trust.

Since much of the Excel functionality has been seen before, we will let you treat much of the rest of this scenario as a revision exercise.

Comparing performance to the rest of the country

There is much data here, and we will simply use a few examples as to how it can be used.

The data for My Own Trust is shown in the following tables. You may want to assemble the sheet yourself, or use the one provided on the website. Either way, the completed sheet is shown at the end of the tables.

Table 1 Hospital Waiting Times	
All specialties 13 weeks	67%
All specialties 26 weeks	95%
Did not attend 1st op app	12%
Wait in outpatient clinic	78%
All specialties 3 months	68%
All specialties 12 months	93%
Action after cancelled op	27%

Table 2 Day case surgery rates	
Inguinal hernia repair	30
Cataract extraction	59
Laparoscopy sterilisation	54

Table 3a&b Waiting times: % of outpatients seen within 13 and 26 weeks

	13 weeks	26 weeks
All specialties	73	97
General surgery	74	100
Urology	88	100
Trauma and orthopaedics	44	100
Ear, nose and throat	46	100
Ophthalmology	74	78
Oral surgery	79	98
Plastic surgery	63	78
Gynaecology	78	89
General medicine	88	93
Dermatology	55	93
Mental illness	88	100
Cardiology	83	98
Paediatrics	95	96
Rheumatology	71	98

Table 4a&b   Waiting times: % of patients admitted within 3 and 12 months

	3 months	12 months
All specialties	66	95
General surgery	63	95
Urology	67	97
Trauma and orthopaedics	37	93
Ear, nose and throat	64	92
Ophthalmology	51	96
Oral surgery	83	100
Plastic surgery	58	87
Gynaecology	83	99
Cardiothoracic surgery		87
Cardiology	97	100
Paediatric surgery	93	98
Paediatrics	78	99
General medicine	95	98
Gastroenterology	50	87

Table 5   Complaints

Total written complaints	567
Local resolution action	491
Independent review	12

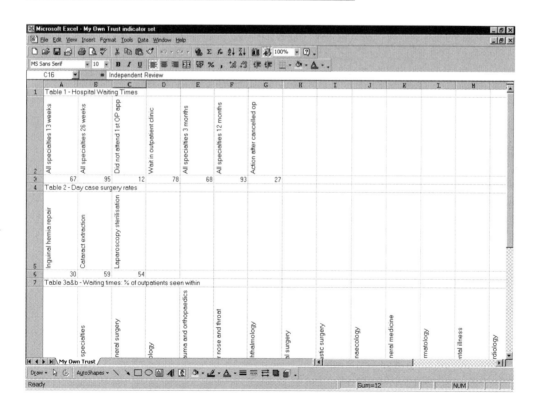

In order to establish our relative performance we will adopt a strategy which can be applied to any of the indicators:

1   describe the overall national distribution of the indicator
2   construct a frequency distribution table for the indicator
3   construct a frequency distribution chart for the indicator
4   order the national indicators.

In each case we then describe our performance relative to national data.

We will take as our example, all specialties seen within 13 weeks.

The national data for this indicator is stored at [National NHS indicator data 1997.xls]ENGL1'!G8:G393.

Health warning

Before we proceed, ensure that both the national data workbook and the My Own Trust data workbooks are open, otherwise nasty VALUE! Error messages may result when Excel cannot find the data it requires to complete a formula.

We will start a new workbook for the analysis of each indicator:

🖰 **Click** on ▯.

On the first sheet we enter the descriptive statistics:

🖰 **Click** on A1

⌨ **Type** %All specialties seen within 13 weeks.

To enter the descriptive statistics:

🖰 **Click** on Tools in the menu bar

🖰 **Click** on Data Analysis in the Tools menu

🖰 **Click** on Descriptive Statistics in the list

🖰 **Click** on ▭ OK ▭

⌨ **Type** '[National NHS indicator data 1997.xls]ENGL1'!$G$8:$G$393 at the Input Range.

> **Hint**
>
>
>
> This range can also be selected by mouse by first clicking on ⊠ at the right-hand end of the range box.
>
> From here, you can select the required workbook, then cell range.

🖱️ **Click** on Output Range

⌨️ **Type** $A$2 to enter the value as the start of the output range

🖱️ **Click** on Summary Statistics.

By now, the dialog box should look something like the one below:

Descriptive Statistics   **? X**

Input
- Input Range: `'[National NHS indica` ⊠
- Grouped By: ⦿ Columns   ○ Rows
- ☐ Labels in First Row

    OK   **Cancel**   **Help**

Output options
- ○ Output Range: ⊠
- ⦿ New Worksheet Ply: `$a$2`
- ○ New Workbook
- ☐ Summary statistics
- ☐ Confidence Level for Mean: `95` %
- ☐ Kth Largest: `1`
- ☐ Kth Smallest: `1`

⌨️ **Click** on ⟦ OK ⟧.

To obtain the result below, I deleted the row (row 3) with the heading supplied by Excel ('Column 1') and widened Column A to twice its original width:

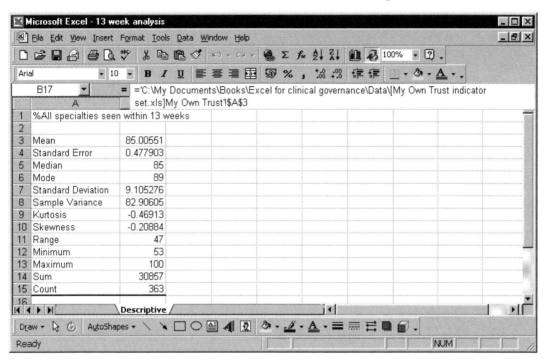

To complete this sheet, we simply add My Own Trust's performance for comparison:

🖰 **Click** on A17

⌨ **Type** Trust Performance

⌨ **Press** [Tab] to move to cell B17

🖰 **Click** on <u>W</u>indow in the menu bar

🖰 **Click** on My Own Trust indicator set

🖰 **Click** on A3 in the Window menu

🖰 **Click** on 🗈

🖰 **Click** on <u>W</u>indow in the menu bar

🖰 **Click** on Book1 in the Window menu

🖰 **Click** on <u>E</u>dit in the menu bar

🖰 **Click** on Paste <u>S</u>pecial in the Edit menu

🖰 **Click** on Paste <u>L</u>ink.

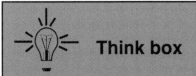

Think box

Looking at this analysis, think about the following questions:

1 what does it mean?
2 is the result a good one for the Trust?
3 does it require action?
4 if so, what might you do?

At this point, it's probably worth saving the sheet as '13 week analysis'. You know how to do this by now!

Next, we will construct a frequency distribution table for this indicator in sheet 2. The above analysis tells us that the minimum value is 53, the maximum is 100, with a mean and median falling at around 85:

🖰   **Click** on the sheet2 tab to move to a blank sheet

🖰   **Click** on A1

⌨   **Type** Value

⌨   **Press** [tab]

⌨   **Type** Freq

⌨   **Press** [tab]

⌨   **Type** Value

⌨   **Press** [tab]

⌨   **Type** Freq

⌨   **Press** ↵

🖰   **Click** on the sheet1 tab to move to the previous analysis

🖰   **Click** on B12 (containing the minimum value)

🖰   **Click** on 📋

🖰   **Click** on the sheet2 tab to return to the second analysis

🖰   **Click** on A2

🖰   **Click** on 📋

⌨   **Press** ↵ to move to A3

⌨ **Type** =A2+1

⌨ **Press** ↵

🖰 **Click** on A3 again

🖰 **AutoFill** down to A49

🖰 **Click** on B2

⌨ **Type** =COUNTIF('[National NHS indicator data 1997.xls]ENGL1'!$G$8:$G$393,A2)

⌨ **Press** ↵.

Hint

This formula says 'count the number of cells in the range G8:G393 in the worksheet ENGL1 in the workbook National NHS indicator data 1997.xls that have the same value as cell A2'.

Aren't you glad I told you that?

🖰 **Click** on B2 again

🖰 **AutoFill** down to A49.

Now to construct our banded frequency table:

🖰 **Click** on C2

⌨ **Type** 50–55

⌨ **Press** ↵

⌨ **Type** 56–60

⌨ **Press** ↵

⌨ **Type** 61–65

⌨ **Press** ↵

⌨ **Type** 66–70

⌨ **Press** ↵

⌨ **Type** 71–75

⌨ **Press** ↵

⌨ **Type** 76–80

⌨ **Press** ↵

⌨ **Type** 81–85

⌨ **Press** ↵

⌨ **Type** 86–90

⌨ **Press** ↵

⌨ **Type** 91–95

⌨ **Press** ↵

⌨ **Type** 96–100

⌨ **Press** ↵

🖱 **Click** on D2.

There are two ways to do the next bit:

Either: Or:

⌨ **Type** =SUM(B2:B4)   ⌨ **Type** =SUM(B2:B4)

⌨ **Press** ↵   ⌨ **Press** ↵

🖱 **AutoFill** down to D11   🖱 **AutoFill** down to D11

🖱 **Click** on D3   🖱 **Click** on D3

⌨ **Edit** the formula to read   🖱 **Highlight** B3:B5 in the formula
=SUM(B5:B9)
                                            🖱 **Highlight** B5:B9 in the worksheet to
                                            update the formula

⌨ **Press** ↵ to accept the new formula   ⌨ **Press** ↵ to accept the new formula
and move to D4   and move to D4

⌨ **Edit** the formula to read   🖱 **Highlight** B4:B6 in the formula
=SUM(B10:B14)
                                            🖱 **Highlight** B10:B14 in the worksheet

⌨ **Press** ↵   ⌨ **Press** ↵

⌨ **Edit** the formula to read   🖱 **Highlight** B5:B7 in the formula
=SUM(B15:B19)
                                            🖱 **Highlight** B15:B19 in the worksheet

⌨ **Press** ↵   ⌨ **Press** ↵

⌨ **Edit** the formula to read   🖱 **Highlight** B6:B8 in the formula
=SUM(B20:B24)

- ⌨ **Press** ↵
- ⌨ **Edit** the formula to read =SUM(B25:B29)
- ⌨ **Press** ↵
- ⌨ **Edit** the formula to read =SUM(B30:B34)
- ⌨ **Press** ↵
- ⌨ **Edit** the formula to read =SUM(B35:B39)
- ⌨ **Press** ↵
- ⌨ **Edit** the formula to read =SUM(B40:B44)
- ⌨ **Press** ↵
- ⌨ **Edit** the formula to read =SUM(B45:B49)
- ⌨ **Press** ↵.

- ⌐ **Highlight** B20:B24 in the worksheet
- ⌨ **Press** ↵
- ⌐ **Highlight** B7:B9 in the formula
- ⌐ **Highlight** B25:B29 in the worksheet
- ⌨ **Press** ↵
- ⌐ **Highlight** B8:B10 in the formula
- ⌐ **Highlight** B30:B34 in the worksheet
- ⌨ **Press** ↵
- ⌐ **Highlight** B9:B11 in the formula
- ⌐ **Highlight** B35:B39 in the worksheet
- ⌐ **Highlight** B10:B12 in the formula
- ⌐ **Highlight** B40:B44 in the worksheet
- ⌨ **Press** ↵
- ⌐ **Highlight** B11:B13 in the formula
- ⌐ **Highlight** B45:B49 in the worksheet
- ⌨ **Press** ↵.

The banded frequency table is now complete.

Exercise

The task of producing a frequency distribution chart in a separate worksheet in the book is left as an exercise.

A model answer is provided overleaf. You may want to try to reproduce this result.

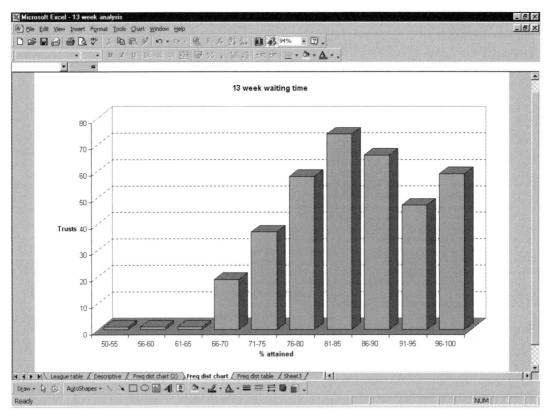

Now we can get really smart and add the Trust performance to the chart.

The first part is revision and is therefore left as an exercise.

Exercise

To help with visibility re-format the background (known as the walls) with no Fill colour and use Format Gridlines to change the gridlines to dashed.

Hint

Remember to use the 🖑 **Right-click** to access the short menus to change features of the graph.

Once these changes have been made, we can then add the Trust's performance at 67% to our chart:

🖰 **Click** on Y̲iew in the menu bar

🖰 **Click** on T̲oolbars in the View menu

🖰 **Click** on Drawing in the sub-menu.

The drawing menu should now appear. We are going to add a vertical line at 67 and a text box as a label and change them both to red:

🖰 **Click** on \ in the drawing toolbar

🖰 **Click** on the point corresponding to 67% at the bottom of the chart at the rear of the appropriate bar

🖰 **Drag** the mouse to the top of the chart so as to draw a vertical line

🖰 **Right-click** on the resulting line

🖰 **Click** on Format Aut̲oshape.

From the Colors and Lines section of the resulting box:

🖰 **Click** on ▾ in the C̲olor box

🖰 **Click** on Red in the resulting options of colours

🖰 **Click** on ▭OK▭ .

Now we add the text box:

🖰 **Click** on ▣ in the drawing toolbar

🖰 **Click** on the chart next to the line

⌨ **Type** Trust Performance

🖰 **Highlight** Trust Performance

🖰 **Click** on ▾ next to the font size in the formatting toolbar

🖰 **Click** on 12 in the resulting list

🖰 **Click** on A̲▾ in the formatting toolbar

🖰 **Click** on Red in the resulting options of colours.

Hopefully, the result will look something like the one below:

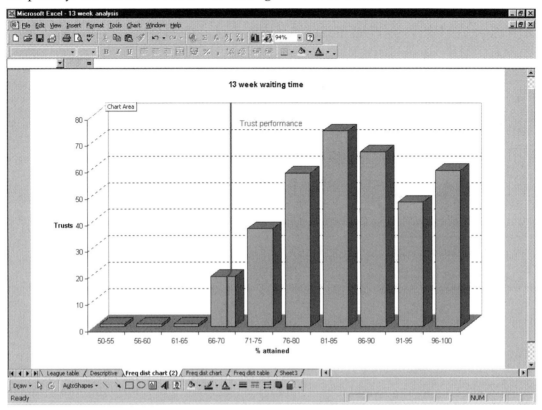

The final analysis is to construct a league table.

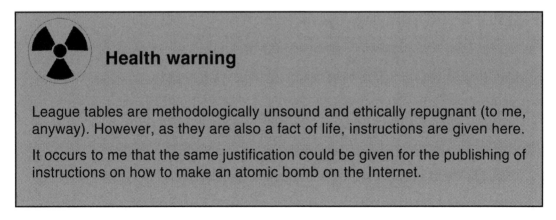

Health warning

League tables are methodologically unsound and ethically repugnant (to me, anyway). However, as they are also a fact of life, instructions are given here.

It occurs to me that the same justification could be given for the publishing of instructions on how to make an atomic bomb on the Internet.

First, we need to copy the basic waiting time data from our national data set. The easiest place to find this data is in the sheet ENGL1 in our national data workbook.

To start, return to the national data workbook:

🖱 **Click** on <u>W</u>indow in the menu bar

🖱 **Click** on National indicator dataset 1997 in the Window menu

🖱 **Click** on the ENGL1 tab at the bottom of the sheets to select this sheet

🖱 **Click** on <u>E</u>dit in the menu bar

🖱 **Click** on <u>M</u>ove or copy sheet

🖱 **Click** on ▾ in the <u>T</u>o book: box

🖱 **Click** on 13 week analysis in the list

🖱 **Click** on <u>C</u>reate a copy

🖱 **Click** on ⟨ OK ⟩ .

🖱 **Select** Columns B to F

🖱 **Click** on <u>E</u>dit in the menu bar

🖱 **Click** on <u>D</u>elete

🖱 **Select** Column C

🖱 **Click** on <u>E</u>dit in the menu bar

🖱 **Click** on <u>D</u>elete

🖱 **Select** Column D to U

🖱 **Click** on Edit in the menu bar

🖱 **Click** on <u>D</u>elete

🖱 **Select** Rows 5 to 7

🖱 **Click** on <u>E</u>dit in the menu bar

🖱 **Click** on <u>D</u>elete.

Now to sort our data into a table:

🖰 **Select** A5 to C390

🖰 **Click** on <u>D</u>ata in the menu bar

🖰 **Click** on <u>S</u>ort

🖰 **Click** on No header ro<u>w</u>

🖰 **Click** on ▾ in the Sort by box

🖰 **Click** on Column B in the list

🖰 **Click** on Descending

🖰 **Click** on ▾ in the Then by box

🖰 **Click** on Column C in the list

🖰 **Click** on Descen<u>d</u>ing.

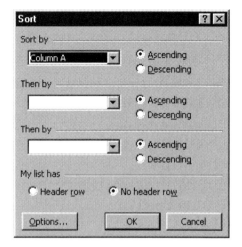

When the box looks like the one opposite:

🖰 **Click** on [OK].

The result is the Trusts sorted in terms of waiting times, percentage of patients seen in under 13 weeks first, then in order of the percentage of patients seen in under 26 weeks where the first fails to distinguish.

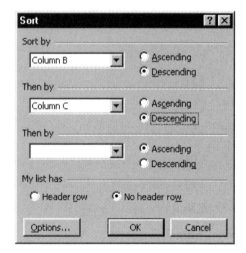

If we want to assign a rank order (ugh!) then the fun begins. The problem arises from those Trusts who have identical performance in terms of these indicators. For example the first 22 Trusts all achieve 100% performance in terms of these indicators.

One way to deal with this is to use a hidden column:

🖰 **Click** on D5

⌨ **Type** 1

⌨ **Press** ↵

⌨ **Type** =D5+1

⌨ **Press** ↵

◌ **Click** on D6

◌ **AutoFill** down to D390.

This is the raw rank order, unable to distinguish identical Trust performances. We now hide this column:

◌ **Select** Column D

◌ **Right-click** in Column D.

From the resulting short menu:

◌ **Click** on Hide.

Now to use this hidden column to assign a true rank order:

◌ **Select** Column A

◌ **Click** on Insert in the menu bar

◌ **Click** on Columns in the Insert menu

◌ **Click** on A4

⌨ **Type** Rank

⌨ **Press** ↵

⌨ **Type** 1

⌨ **Press** ↵

⌨ **Type** =IF(C5=C6,IF(D5=D6,A5,E5),E5)

◌ **Click** on A6

⌨ **AutoFill** down to A390.

This table puts My Own Trust at about 354th in the league table!

Hint

In plain English, this formula says if the values for this Trust are identical to the one above it, give it the same rank order, otherwise use the raw score from the hidden column (which has become E since we inserted a new column to accommodate true rank order).

Exercise

To tidy this up, we should rename the sheets appropriately:

1 rename ENGL1 as League table

2 rename Sheet1 as Descriptive

3 rename Chart1 as Freq dist chart

4 rename Sheet2 as Freq dist table

Think box

Now that you have considered four different ways of analysing your performance.

• Which is the most helpful?

• Which is the most likely to induce change?

Exercise

Produce a similar analysis based on the My Own Trust data for the following clinical specialties:

1 general surgery

2 ear, nose and throat

3 gynaecology

Model answers are provided on the website.

Exercise

Find the data for your local Trust in the national data, and repeat the 13 week analysis for your local Trust.

This time you're on your own – no model answers are provided on the website.

Apologies to readers in Wales, Scotland and elsewhere – pick yourself a Trust at random or try to track down comparable data.

Risk management in patient care

In this chapter

This chapter will tell you how to:

- consider relative risk in patient management

- use risk management techniques or predict risk

- use techniques already seen to predict risk

- apply corrections for small samples in chi-squared test

- make use of existing evidence to avoid the use of horrendously complex statistics that most of us couldn't use properly anyway!

 calculate relative risks and confidence limits

 apply a correction to chi-squared tests for small samples in Excel.

Risk management is not in fact new in healthcare, although many clinicians may find it so. It has traditionally been used widely in public health and to manage population-wide health issues. Under clinical governance, it is likely to be brought explicitly into the care of individuals as part of the evidence base on which decisions about care are made. However, it is important to realise that it deals in probabilities, not certainties, and it is important to recognise the uncertainty associated with any calculations.

It is also worth noting that the techniques required by many risk management scenarios are not fundamentally different from those already seen. In other cases, due to the multiplicity of risk factors operating, it is unreasonable to expect non-specialists to carry out full analyses. In all cases, it is important to recognise the limitations of the analyses carried out.

We will use a series of mini-scenarios to show how practising clinicians can use published evidence to evaluate relative risks for their patients, which is the obligation placed upon them by clinical governance.

Scenario 1

Your practice has adopted a policy of promoting the use of aspirin to all patients considered to be at risk from hypertension. One of your colleagues has raised the issue of patients suffering from pregnancy-induced hypertension during the third trimester of pregnancy.

A search of Medline reveals a study from 1989 by Schiff *et al.*[1] In the study, 65 patients participated in the trial. 34 were given 100mg of aspirin daily, the remainder were given a matching placebo.

The results were as follows

	Aspirin	*Placebo*	*Total*
Hypertension	4	11	15
No hypertension	30	20	50
Total	34	31	65

First, we build a simple summary table in a new Excel sheet.

Start a new workbook:

🖱 **Click** on ⬜ in the tool bar

🖱 **Click** on B1

⌨ **Type** Aspirin

⌨ **Press** [tab]

⌨ **Type** Placebo

⌨ **Press** [tab]

[1] Schiff E, Peleg E, Goldenberg M *et al.* (1989) The use of aspirin to prevent pregnancy-induced hypertension and lower the ratio of thromboxane A_2 to prostacyclin in relatively high risk pregnancies. *NEJM.* **321**: 351–6.

☷ **Type** Total

☷ **Press** ⏎

☷ **Press** [Home] to move to start of line (A2)

Hint

There are a whole load of useful keyboard shortcuts to help you move around. Here are some:

☷ **Press** [Home] to move to start of line

☷ **Press** [Ctrl] and [Home] together to move to the top of the page (A1)

☷ **Press** [Page Down] to move to the first row invisible below the bottom of the page.

☷ **Press** [Page Up] to move to the first row invisible above the top of the page.

These correspond closely to analogous functions in Word.

☷ **Type** Hypertension

☷ **Press** [tab]

☷ **Type** 4

☷ **Press** [tab]

☷ **Type** 11

☷ **Press** [tab]

🖰 **Click** on Σ in the toolbar

☷ **Press** ⏎ to accept the formula

☷ **Press** [Home] to move to start of line (A3)

☷ **Type** No hypertension

☷ **Press** [tab]

☷ **Type** 30

☷ **Press** [tab]

🖮 **Type** 20

🖮 **Press** [tab]

🖱 **Click** on Σ in the toolbar

🖮 **Press** ↵ to accept the formula

🖮 **Press** [Home] to move to A4

🖮 **Type** Total

🖮 **Press** [tab]

🖱 **Click** on Σ in the toolbar

🖮 **Press** [tab] to accept the formula

🖮 **Press** [⇧] and [tab] together to move back to B4

🖱 **AutoFill** across to D4.

By now, your table should look like the one shown above, or in the Excel sheet below:

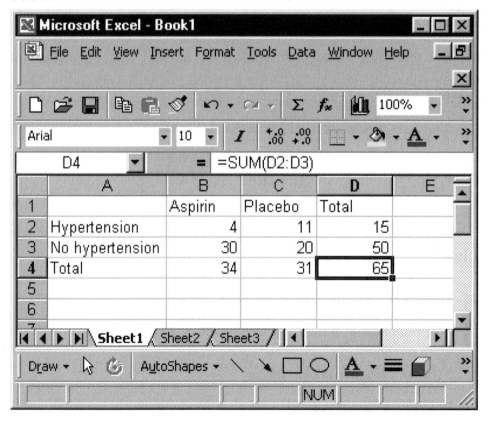

The simplest measure of relative risk is given by the relative proportions:

 Click on A5

Type Proportion

Press [tab]

Type =B2/B4

 AutoFill across to C5

 Highlight B5 and C5

 Click on (decrease decimal) in the toolbar until two decimal places are showing.

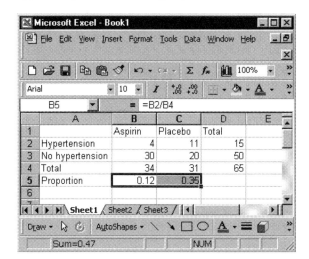

 ## Principle of good practice

All of the techniques discussed in this scenario are approximations. It is always good practice to reduce the number of decimal places shown to an appropriate level of significance.

Whilst this has the merit of simplicity, we need to assess the confidence we can have in this result. We can do this in two ways.

Previously, we have seen how to carry out a chi-squared test to measure the probability of an association.

Exercise

Use a chi-squared test to evaluate the probability of an association between the administration of aspirin and the occurrence of hypertension in this group of patients, using the CHITEST function as before.

The end result is shown below.

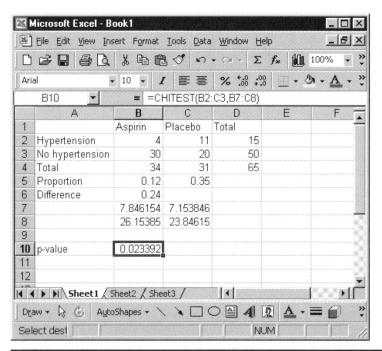

The p-value looks significant, but see the **Health warning** below!

Health warning

Chi-squared calculations are inaccurate at small sample sizes. This arises because the chi-squared test assumes a continuous distribution, and at small sample sizes, this is increasingly inaccurate. A number of corrections are available for this. Among the best known are the Yates correction, which can be applied 2 x 2 tables, and the Fisher exact test, which is computationally more complex, but more generally applicable.

Of these, the Yates correction is easier to calculate without a specialist statistics package, so its use will be shown here.

Hint

The ,1 in the CHIDIST function refers to the degrees of freedom. In this case this is the number of independent variables – in this case one.

Hint

To carry out the Yates corrected test, we must dig a bit into the theory of the chi-squared test.

In a conventional chi-squared test we calculate a chi value shown in the proper textbooks as χ^2 (literally chi-squared). Traditionally, we have then looked up in a table the probability value (p) which corresponds to this chi-squared value. (If you want to know how this is calculated, then you need at least a statistics book, better a statistician and preferably a very strong cup of coffee or stronger stimulant.)

So far we have got Excel to do all the work for us, using the CHITEST function. This function takes the actual and expected value tables and does two steps in one:

1 calculates the corresponding χ^2 value.
2 translates this into a p-value which it puts into the spreadsheet.

To do this it calculates χ^2 using the following formula:

$$\chi^2 = \frac{N(ad-bc)^2}{(a+b)(a+c)(b+d)(c+d)}$$

where the letters are defined as follows:

	Column 1	Column 2	Total
Row 1	a	b	a+b
Row 2	c	d	c+d
Total	a+c	b+d	N

To apply the Yates correction to correct for this bias we apply a different formula:

$$\chi^2_y = \frac{N(|ad-bc|-(N/2))^2}{(a+b)(a+c)(b+d)(c+d)}$$

In Excel we must calculate the Yates χ^2_y value using first principles.

Fortunately, Excel does provide a function CHIDIST() to turn our modified χ^2_y value into a p-value.

This is the method we will use here:

☝ **Click** on A11

⌨ **Type** |ad-bc|-(N/2)

⌨ **Press** [tab]

⌨ **Type** =ABS((B2*C3)-(C2*B3))-(D4/2)

⌨ **Press** ↵

⌨ **Press** [Home] to move to A12

⌨ **Type** Ordinator

⌨ **Press** [tab]

⌨ **Type** =D4*B11*B11

⌨ **Press** ↵

⌨ **Press** [Home] to move to A13

⌨ **Type** Denominator

⌨ **Press** [tab]

⌨ **Type** =D2*D3*B4*C4

⌨ **Press** ↵

⌨ **Press** [Home] to move to A14

⌨ **Type** Yates Chi value

⌨ **Press** [tab]

⌨ **Type** =B12/B13

⌨ **Press** ↵

⌨ **Press** [Home] to move to A15

⌨ **Type** Yates p value

⌨ **Press** [tab]

⌨ **Type** =CHIDIST(B14,1)

⌨ **Press** ↵.

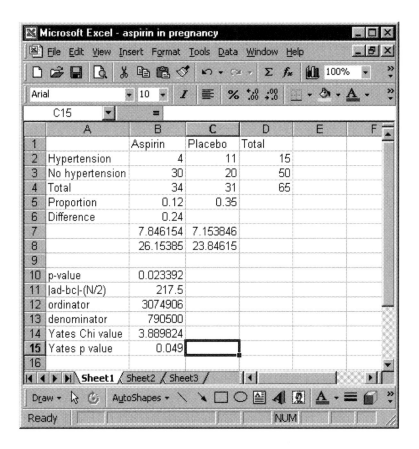

There is an alternative way to consider whether findings are significant. Increasingly, findings are being quoted with confidence limits, often 95% confidence limits. This is good practice and should be adopted where possible.

We can calculate 95% confidence limits for this example, but first we add a cell to calculate the difference in proportions:

🖱 **Click** on B6

⌨ **Type** =C5–B5.

The answer should be 0.24. At the bottom of our sheet, we will calculate the confidence limits associated with this difference.

WWW For those who found the previous section hard going, a shortcut is provided on the accompanying website. From here you can download a generalised calculator of the Yates corrected χ^2_y and p-values. This allows you to enter data for any 2x2 trial and calculate corrected and uncorrected results.

Exercise

The above calculator was constructed from the example in the text, and merely uses the formatting commands seen previously.

The more adventurous reader may like to construct their own!

Hint

The 95% confidence limits are calculated from the standard error. The standard error of the difference between the observed proportions, p_1-p_2 :

$$se\ (p_1\text{-}p_2) = \sqrt{var(p_1)\text{-}\ var(p_2)}$$

where $var(p_i) = \dfrac{p_i\ (1\text{-}\ p_i)}{n_i}$

The upper and lower confidence limits are given by:

$$(p_1\text{-}p_2) \pm 1.96 \times se(p_1\text{-}p_2)$$

NB: This assumes a Normal sampling distribution – see a statistician for more details, and in practice avoid small samples!

🖰 **Click** on A17

⌨ **Type** var(p1)

⌨ **Press** [tab]

⌨ **Type** =(B5*(1-B5))/B4

⌨ **Press** ⏎

⌨ **Press** [Home]

⌨ **Type** var(p2)

⌨ **Press** [tab]

⌨ **Type** =(C5*(1-C5))/C4

⌨ **Press** ⏎

⌨ **Press** [Home]

⌨ **Type** Standard error

⌨ **Press** [tab]

⌨ **Type** =SQRT(B17+B18)

⌨ **Press** ⏎

⌨ **Press** [Home]

⌨ **Type** Lower 95% limit

⌨ **Press** [tab]

⌨ **Type** =B6-(1.96*B19)

⌨ **Press** ⏎

⌨ **Press** [Home]

⌨ **Type** Lower 95% limit

⌨ **Press** [tab]

⌨ **Type** =B6+(1.96*B19)

⌨ **Press** ⏎

⌨ **Press** [Home]

⌨ **Highlight** B17 to B21

🖰 **Click** on 🔢 (decrease decimal) in the toolbar until four decimal places are showing.

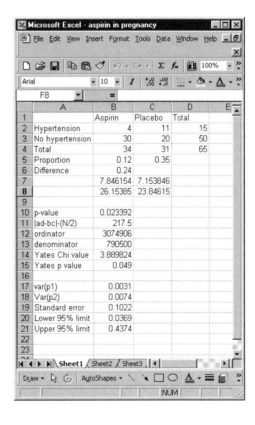

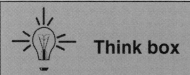

Think box

This analysis shows a corrected p-value of 0.049 and wide confidence limits of 0.037 to 0.44 for the difference in proportions.

Think about the following questions:

1 how confident can you be in this treatment?
2 what other factors might also need to be taken into account in a clinical decision?
3 what might you do as a consequence?

Scenario 2

In our second case, we look at the management of smoking among patients and seek to develop a risk ready-reckoner to assist in the targeting of intensive counselling.

We have identified our target population of 5650 males, aged 40–59, across our PCG.

The following factors are reckoned to influence the probability that patients would abstain from smoking for 6 months:

- number of years smoking cigarettes
- mean blood pressure
- diagnosis of ischaemic heart disease
- angina
- family history of fatal heart problems
- diabetes.

The purpose of the score is to find a way of combining these factors and defining a weighting.

The approach we will use is based upon a study by Shaper et al.[2]

In the original study, logistic regression was used to calculate co-efficients for weighting the different factors. From their analysis of 7056 men, they calculated

[2] Shaper AG, Pocock SJ, Phillips AN and Walker M (1986) Identifying men at risk of heart attacks: strategy for use in general practice. *BMJ.* **293**: 474–9.

weightings derived from the logistic regression analysis, and normalised them so that the men at the eightieth percentile scored 1000.

It is beyond the scope of Excel to reproduce the original analysis. More importantly, it is beyond the scope of the author to explain it in such a way that the reader could reproduce it reliably.

Therefore, we will adopt an alternative simplified strategy which we believe is more appropriate for the clinicians. This consists of three steps:

1   identify the best evidence available for your problem
2   use their weightings to calculate a risk
3   normalise your population to take account of local variations.

Health warning

All risk assessment is a predictive forecast. It is therefore a 'guesstimate'. Our job is to produce the best 'guesstimate' possible within the constraints available. The constraints may include base data, IT and statistical skills as well as that old perennial, time and money.

The Shaper study produced a risk score based upon the following formula:

Risk =

- 7 x years smoking +
- 6.5 x mean blood pressure (mmHg) +
- 270 if the man recalls a diagnosis of ischaemic heart disease +
- 150 if there was evidence of angina +
- 85 if either patient had died of heart trouble +
- 150 if he was diabetic.

The data from the target population across our PCG can be found in the workbook heart risk data.xls:

🖰   **Open** heart risk data.xls.

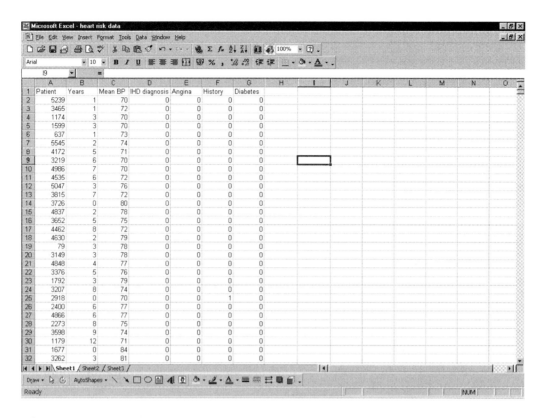

The file contains data on 5650 patients.

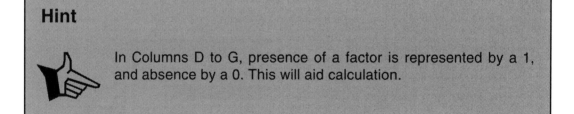

Hint

In Columns D to G, presence of a factor is represented by a 1, and absence by a 0. This will aid calculation.

Our first job is to calculate a raw risk score based upon the Shaper weightings:

🖱 **Click** on H1

⌨ **Type** Raw scores

⌨ **Press** ↵

⌨ **Type** =(B2*7)+(C2*6.5)+(D2*270)+(E2*150)+(F2*85)+(G2*150)

⌨ **Press** ↵

⌨ **Press** [Up Arrow]

🖱 **AutoFill** down to H5651.

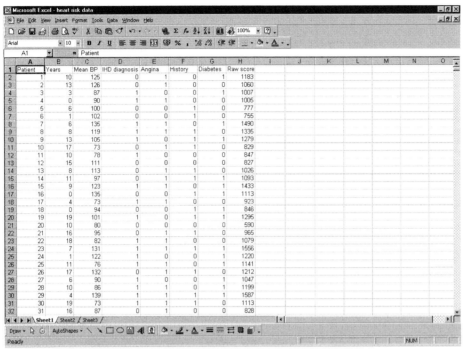

The next step is to normalise the scores so that for our local population, the highest risk 20% of patients are scored at 1000 or more to take account of overall population differences between those in the Shaper study and those in our PCG.

First, we calculate a rank order. To do this, we sort the data on the raw score column:

🖱 **Highlight** Columns A to H

🖱 **Click** on Data in the menu bar

🖱 **Click** on Sort in the data menu

🖱 **Click** on ▼ in the Sort by box

🖱 **Click** on Raw Score in the resulting list

🖱 **Click** on OK .

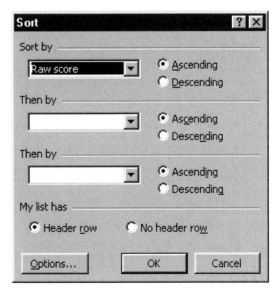

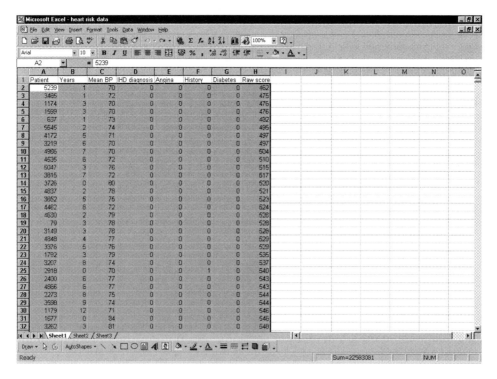

The patients are now ranked in risk order. To assign a ranking:

🖰 **Click** on I1

⌨ **Type** Ranking

⌨ **Press** ↵

⌨ **Type** 1

⌨ **Press** ↵

⌨ **Type** =I2+1

⌨ **Press** ↵

⌨ **Press** [Up Arrow]

🖰 **AutoFill** down to I5651.

Now to convert it to a centile:

🖰 **Click** on J1

⌨ **Type** Centile

⌨ **Press** ↵

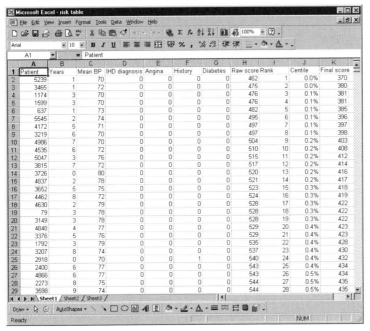

Type =I2/I$5651

Press ↵

Press [Up Arrow]

AutoFill down to J5651

Highlight Column J

Click on % in the tool bar

Click on [icon] to add one decimal place.

By a happy coincidence, the eightieth centile falls at 1250 on our raw scores. This means that the normalisation process consists of multiplying our raw scores by 0.8.

Click on K1

Type Final score

Press ↵

Type =J2*0.8

Press ↵

Press [Up Arrow]

AutoFill down to K5651.

Think box

Think about the following questions:

1 how valid is this kind of analysis?
2 what assumptions are we making?
3 is there a better way?
4 is any proposed alternative solution feasible and cost-effective
5 is it good enough to use in practice?

Getting data from your proprietary system and into Excel

In this chapter

This chapter will:

- extract data from your proprietary system

- discuss the relevance of MIQUEST

 tell you how to import data into Excel.

Converting data from the proprietary patient record systems into PC applications for analysis has been a perennial problem for the NHS in England and Wales. This topic is dealt with in much more detail in *Information and IT for Primary Care.*

So as not to stop you buying that book, we confine ourselves here to a single fairy story (the aforementioned book has more of them) before moving on to some solutions.

---

[1] Gillies AC (1999) *Information and IT for Primary Care: everything you need to know but are afraid to ask.* Radcliffe Medical Press, Oxford.

Once upon a time ...

I was invited to a hospital in the North of England to speak to a meeting of consultants under the title 'What computers can do for you'. They were very interested in the series of demonstrations of PC applications presented to them on the then huge 21" monitor hired for the occasion.

However, each demonstration was punctuated with 'Well, of course, the problem is that we can't get our data off the hospital patient records system and onto a PC'.

I suggested that they contact their Information Department but was assured that it was impossible. After 90 minutes of demos and continuous 'Well of course, the problem is...' interruptions, I dismantled the kit and carried the hernia-inducing monitor down the stairs.

As I'm packing the brute of a monitor into my car, I'm met by one of the attendees, who greets me and says 'I don't know what they are talking about, I've been getting data off the system for 18 months'. Not that he'd bothered to inform the meeting you understand!

Of course, this is only a fairy story (allegedly!); something so ridiculous couldn't happen in real life could it? It illustrates the fact that the problems with data exchange are human and organisational ones. The barriers to data collection over the last 10 years have been largely ideological and commercial rather than technical.

Happily, things have changed somewhat over the last few years. It is now possible to extract information from many clinical systems including the three most recent from EMIS, In Practice Systems and AAH Meditel.

We will consider first a general strategy and then consider the specific cases of how to extract data from these three systems. Finally, we illustrate the use of the MIQUEST software, which has arrived a little too late to be of maximum use.

A general strategy

The general strategy is made up of a number of steps:

1 generate a report in the proprietary system
2 export the output as a comma separated text file
3 import the text file into Excel, or other 'open' application.

The comma separated file is a text file and represents a basic format which can be produced and read by many different systems.

The following spreadsheet was taken from the very first scenario:

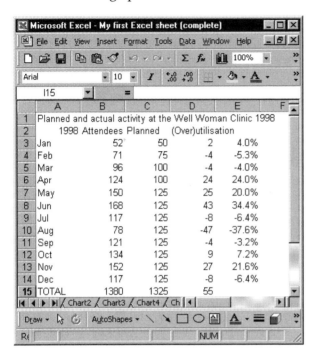

This data can be represented as a comma separated file, shown below:

Planned and actual activity at the Well Woman Clinic 1998,,,,,,,,
1998,Attendees,Planned,(Over)utilisation,,,,
Jan,52,50,2,4.0%,,,
Feb,71,75,–4,–5.3%,,,
Mar,96,100,–4,–4.0%,,,
Apr,124,100,24,24.0%,,,
May,150,125,25,20.0%,,,
Jun,168,125,43,34.4%,,,
Jul,117,125,–8,–6.4%,,,
Aug,78,125,–47,–37.6%,,,
Sep,121,125,–4,–3.2%,,,
Oct,134,125,9,7.2%,,,
Nov,152,125,27,21.6%,,,
Dec,117,125,-8,-6.4%,,,
TOTAL,1380,1325,55,,,,

These files can be read not only by Excel, but also by databases such as Access or specialist packages such as SPSS.

We now consider how to extract the data file from each of the main systems.

Exporting data from EMIS into Excel using LV

(Contributed by Dr Nick Lowe, General Practitioner, Holland House Medical Centre, Lytham, Lancashire.)

 Health warning

Data security and the Data Protection Act need to be considered when transferring any information from the system by any method, and it is better to avoid using any individual patient identifiers in the data unless data security can be guaranteed.

This is further discussed in *Information and IT for Primary Care*.

The EMIS system used in primary care in the UK contains sophisticated search and reporting facilities that can be greatly enhanced by using the powerful features of a spreadsheet such as Excel.

Search and audit results are normally viewed as text on paper printouts but it is easy to export such results into a spreadsheet for further manipulation. Using EMIS with Excel provides a powerful method of analysing and presenting clinical data in a variety of ways for use either by the practice or PCG. This can be a great help with practice audits and will be increasingly important as clinical governance becomes established.

There are alternative techniques for exporting data from EMIS either as ASCII or Excel files. This depends upon the age and configuration of a practice computer system. Older systems require the work to be done at the main server using a floppy disk for data transfer to another computer, or by using KERMIT software on a PC. Although these methods work well they are more complicated – the use of LV software (free from EMIS) is both quicker and easier, and is the recommended method. This is the method described below.

Most practices now have one or more PCs attached to the clinical system and it is best to export the data using one of these machines as an alternative to the main server. It is even possible to use LV on a PC outside the practice using a modem to export the data into Excel, e.g. direct to a PC at home. Data can then be extracted for use in spreadsheets other than Excel.

Familiarity with the software improves with repeated use and it is better to first try some simple searches and exports to Excel.

The following method is simple to apply but assumes the use of:

- a practice system running EMIS version 4 or 5
- a PC connected to the clinical system using LV software
- a copy of Excel loaded on that same PC
- a working knowledge of the EMIS system including the search and statistics module

The methodology is simple.

Ensure LV software has Excel defined as its default spreadsheet

Run LV and on the menu bar click down 'Settings', then 'Advanced'.

In the spreadsheet section of the window click 'find'. Type EXCEL.EXE in the 'search for' box and click 'find' again. The system will then locate the Excel program. Highlight the directory line in the window and click 'select', then 'close'. This now allows LV to run Excel.

Build and run the required search in EMIS

From the main menu type ST, B, A to build a new search. Choose the directory to store search, construct the search parameters and run the search in the usual way. The search result is a simple list of patients – various aspects of this group can then be looked at in more detail. The methods are explained fully in the EMIS manuals.

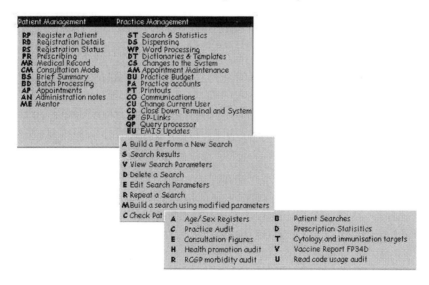

Go to EMIS search results menu and use 'export to Excel' option

From the main menu type ST, B, S and choose option S: 'Search results'.

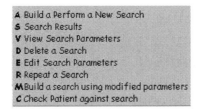

Find the performed search in the directory, select the search line and hit return. This brings up the results output menu. Choose option H 'export results to ASCII file or direct to Excel'.

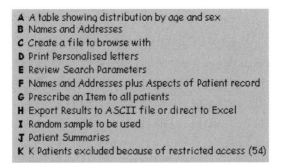

The system then offers the option to change the delimiter character for the data. Leave as ~ (tilde) - the default.

Press return. This brings up the next menu allowing the selection of features to be included in the spreadsheet for those patients identified in the search.

Selecting Aspects Of A Patients Record	
A Registration details	**B** Registration Status
C Diary or Recall Dates	**D** Clinical Aspects of Record
E Present Medication	**F** Past Medication
G Patient Number	**H** GP National Code
I Consultations	**P** Problem Titles
J Age	**T** Temporary Number
S Stored Aspects of Record	**K** Delete Stored Aspects

The menu shows the available options for inclusion in the spreadsheet. For example, if you had performed a search for all the diabetics in the practice you can now gather further details about that group, e.g. option J: Age, option G: Patient Number, and most importantly option D: 'Clinical aspects of Record' – the Read codes, e.g. blood glucose result. A list of features can now be built for export. Medication information is handled better by EMIS version 5.

For each Read code, the associated aspects can be selected according to the filter menu below:

```
         Which of the following to include in the display ?

Earliest date                    : 01.01.1900
Latest date                      : 22.09.1999
Include only latest   (Y/N)      : N
Code description (Y/N)            : Y
Read code (Y/N)                  : N
Date of entry (Y/N)              : Y
Associated features (Y/N)        : N
Associated text (Y/N)            : N
Numerical value (Y/N)            : N
```

Option P for 'Problem Titles' allows additional selections for the inclusion of clinical problem codes recorded in the patient record.

```
Earliest date                                    : 01.01.1900
Latest date                                      : 22.09.1999
Include only latest   (Y/N)                      : N
Code description (Y/N)                            : Y
Read code (Y/N)                                  : N
Date of entry (Y/N)                              : Y
Episode type text (First,review etc) (Y/N)       : █
Place of consultation ? (Y/N)                    :
Consulting doctor (Y/N)                          :
Episode type code (F,N,O) (Y/N)                  :
```

Once all the required aspects have been selected, press return. You are then asked if the features are correct and whether you wish to store the selected aspects for future use – this can be useful if the export is needed again for future comparison or for use with another search group.

In this way a comprehensive selection of data can be compiled for any group identified by a search.

The LV software converts the data and displays the finished spreadsheet in Excel

On pressing return the next menu appears, offering two options. Choose option E: 'export to Excel' and sit back.

A spool file is created – the transfer's progress is displayed on screen and Excel is automatically launched displaying the newly created spreadsheet.

Now you can use the techniques outlined elsewhere in this book to tidy, organise and present the data.

Rename and save the spreadsheet as an Excel file on to disk

The file created will be named by default as stew.csv or similar – this should be renamed and saved to disk as an Excel file with an appropriate filename.

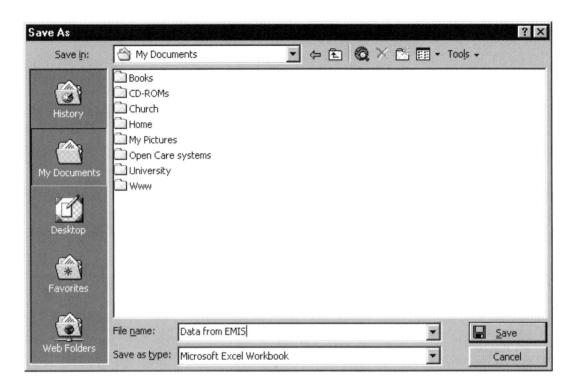

Generating a comma separated text file in In Practice Systems Vision:

(Contributed by Bev Ellis, Practice Manager, Ash Tree House Surgery, Kirkham, Lancashire. The contributor would like to acknowledge the help and support of Alison Young and Hildegard Franke for their invaluable assistance in compiling this section.)

In order to extract a comma separated file, start from the searches and reports main screen in Vision:

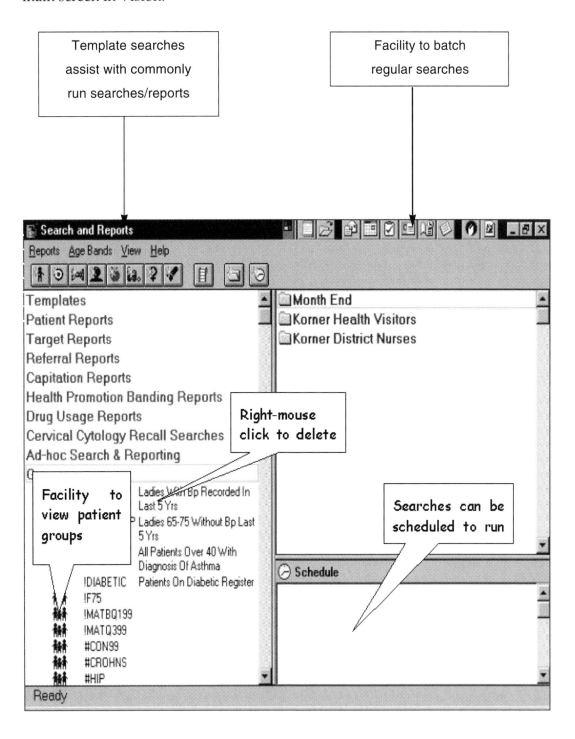

The report module can be used to provide a variety of report outputs. Formats can either be saved for transfer to a spreadsheet package at the output stage, or directly after viewing the results on screen by selecting an option at the end of the viewed results:

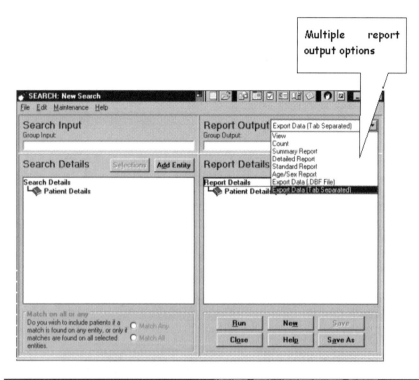

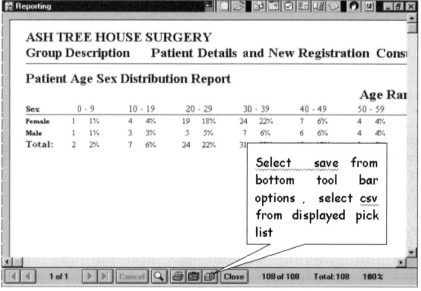

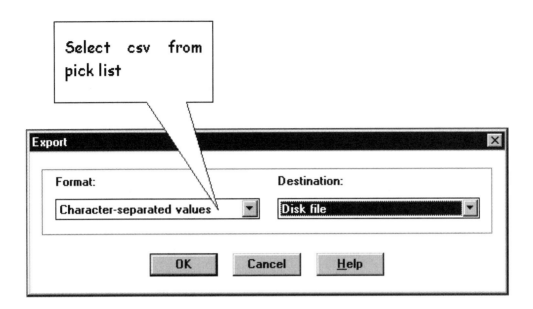

A further option box then presents, enquiring on the type of character separation required, e.g. comma:

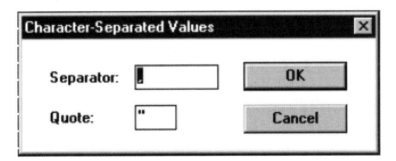

Further options are provided to enable the user to control the output:

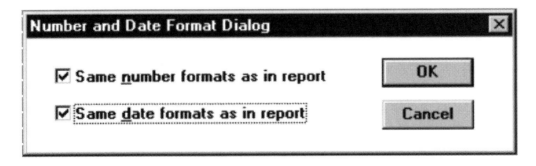

The next step is to open Excel and the file from Vision, e.g. agesex.chr.

The text wizard presents a stepped approach – unfamiliar words such as delimiters simply describe how your data is separated:

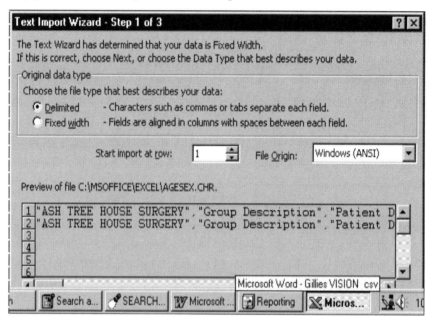

As you can see, the data requires some further manipulation for use within a spreadsheet. The characters that separate the data fields are commas and, therefore, the next step is to insert that information in the selection delimiter field:

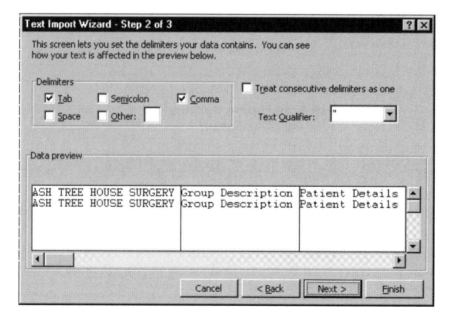

When the finish button is selected, your data is displayed in Excel:

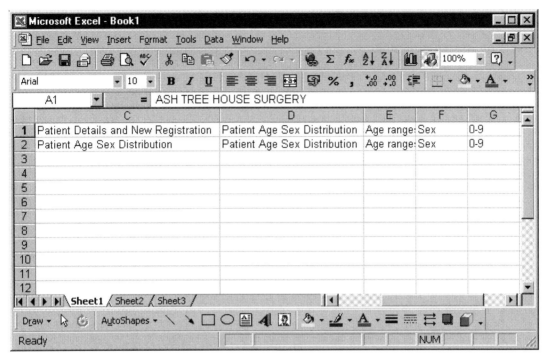

With some further manipulation your data can then be displayed in an appropriate format, e.g. graphs, as described elsewhere:

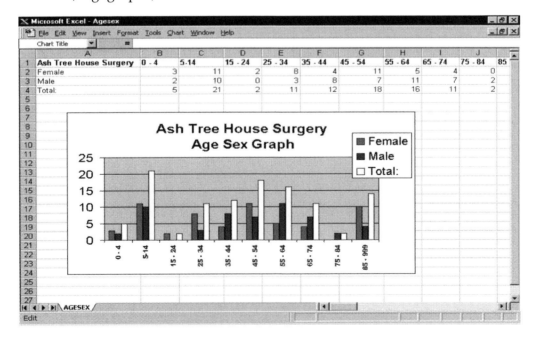

Generating a comma separated text file in Meditel System 6000

(Contributed by Dr Nick Savage, Regent House Surgery, Chorley.)

In order to produce an age–sex register from Meditel 6000 to use in Excel, you need to do the following in System 6000:

- **Open** the S6 Report Manager
- **Open** the folder 'CUSTOM: user defined reports'
- **Open** the folder 'QUICKQRY: Quick query folder'
- **Click** on the 'Add a report' button on the button bar at the top
- **Type** a name for the report, e.g. Agesex
- **Press** ↵
- **Click** 'Yes' to add a new query
- **Click** on 'New Blank Query'
- **Type** a name for the query file
- **Press** ↵
- **Click** on OK
- **Click** 'Yes' to edit the query.

At the query builder window:

- **Type** a meaningful name for the query, e.g. age-sex register
- **Click** the 'New line button'
- **Click** the down arrow to the right of the highlighted 'and' to produce a drop down menu
- **Click** on 'print agesex' in the menu
- **Click** on the 'close' button back at the top
- **Click** on 'yes' to save changes.

The newly created query should be highlighted in the report manager browser.

- **Click** on 'Run query' in the bottom corner.

This will create a csv file called:
C:\MEDDATA\S6000\REPORT\CUSTOM\QUICKQRY\AGESEX.

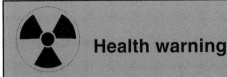

Health warning

Unfortunately, the crude data is presented as numbers of patients in 5 year age bands, e.g. 0–4, 5–9, 10–14 etc, and alternates between males and females for each age band.

To read the comma separated file into Excel

To read the comma separated file into Excel, we simply modify our usual file opening procedure. The file is of a different type and may not be in our usual directory. For example, the MIQUEST report is located on my hard disk under the name 'miquest.txt' in a directory called 'Documents'

In Excel:

🖱 **Click** on 📂 in the tool bar.

First ensure that you are in the correct directory:

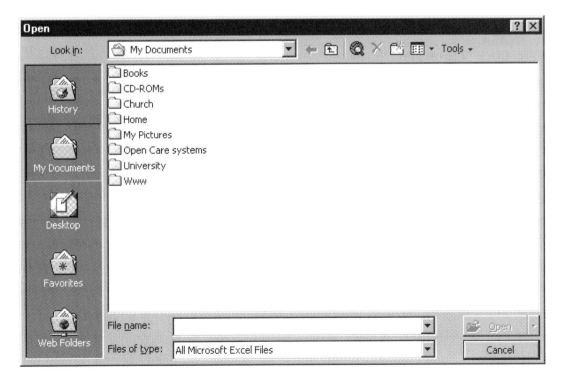

The file will not yet be showing as the box only lists Excel files.

🖱 **Click** on ▼ in the Files of type box.

From the resulting list:

🖱 **Click** on All Files.

The file called 'miquest' should now be visible:

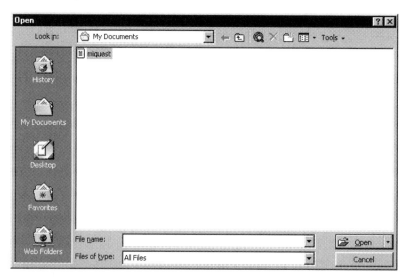

🖱 **Click** on miquest

🖱 **Click** on OK .

The text import Wizard now appears to make life easier (Ha! Ha!).

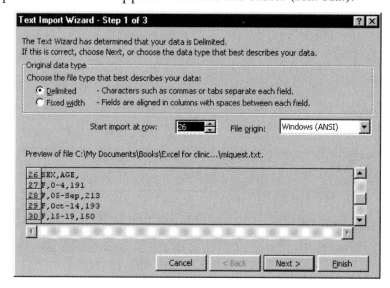

🖰 **Click** on <u>D</u>elimited

🖰 **Click** on Start import at <u>r</u>ow box

⌨ **Press** [Backspace]

⌨ **Type** 26

Hint

Selecting row 26 as the starting point for the import, strips the query from the head of the sheet.

The last two steps are largely for cosmetic purposes and can be omitted without serious damage. If in doubt, repeat the process after completion without these steps.

🖰 **Click** on Next>

🖰 **Click** on <u>C</u>omma as the delimiting character.

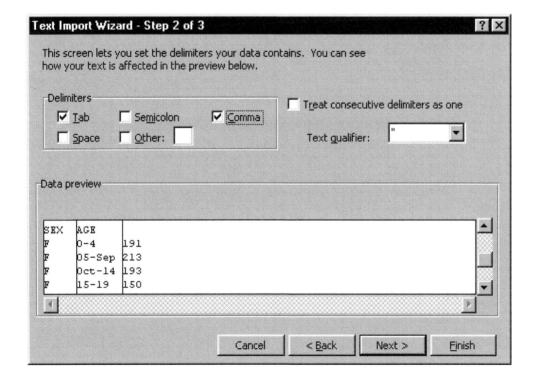

In an attempt to confuse you, Excel decides that the age ranges 5–9 and 10–14 are actually dates. You can attempt to resolve this confusion as follows:

🖱 **Click** on Next>

🖱 **Click** on the Age column

🖱 **Click** on Text.

This should give Excel enough information.

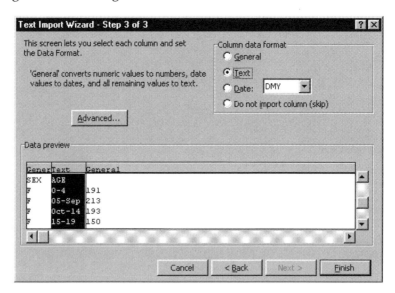

🖱 **Click** on Finish.

But oh dear it doesn't!

The computer thinks it knows best. The question we want to know the answer to is: 'why did it bother to ask us what was in the second column if it was going to ignore it anyway?'

Hint

Further investigation reveals that Excel has already converted the data to a date. So what you have is the text version of the date. If you omit Step 3 by **clicking** on Finish at Step 2 you end up with the date version. Confused? So is the computer.

Read on, it's relatively easy to solve.

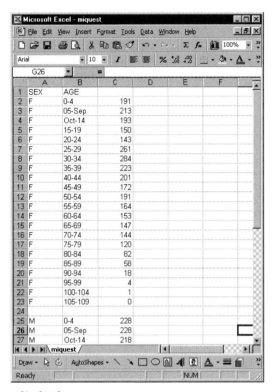

In order to correct Excel's little tantrum:

🖱 **Click** on B3

⌨ **Type** 5–9

⌨ **Press** ↵

⌨ **Type** 10–14.

The sheet is now correct.

Whatever your source and means of importing (EMIS, Meditel etc) it is quite likely that you will need to do a little bit of editing, but it's a lot less than typing it all in again.

From here, the sheet can be treated as a normal sheet. However, it is good practice to save the sheet in Excel format immediately:

🖱 **Click** on 🖫 in the tool bar

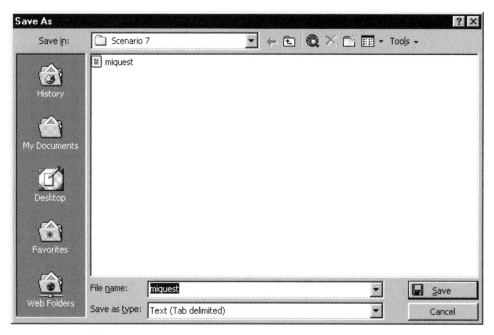

🖰 **Click** on 🔽 in the Save as type box.

From the resulting list:

🖰 **Click** on Microsoft Excel Workbook

🖰 **Click** on File name

⌨ **Type** Imported data or some more suitable name

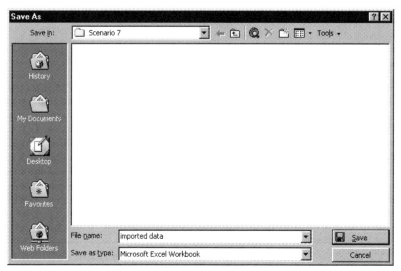

🖰 **Click** on Save.

MIQUEST

The proposed official solution to data extraction is MIQUEST. MIQUEST is a combination of a software tool to overcome the technical barriers and a set of procedural guidelines to allay fears over confidentiality.

The technical part of MIQUEST is a query language and an interpreter. The query language is funnily enough a language in which you write queries. An example of a query would be 'how many patients have had a heart attack in the last year?'.

Schematically, we can think of MIQUEST as laid out below:[2]

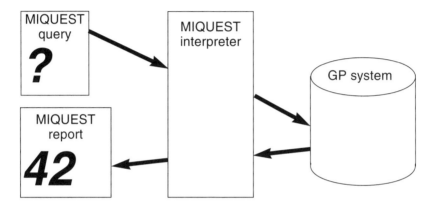

The second part of MIQUEST is the MIQUEST data collection protocol which contain full data security and confidentiality safeguards.

Safeguards specified by MIQUEST protocols

Before a query is run, the practice has:
- the opportunity to scrutinise the query
- the necessity of authorising the query before it can be run
- the safeguard that an external enquirer, e.g. a data collection scheme, may not access any strong patient identifiers, such as names, addresses, full dates of birth, full postcode etc.

After a query has been run, the practice has:
- the opportunity to scrutinise the response
- the necessity of authorising the response before it is released to the enquirer.

[2] In *The Hitch Hiker's Guide to the Galaxy* (Pan Books, 1978) Deep Thought claims that 42 is the answer to the ultimate question of Life, the Universe and everything. Apologies to younger readers!

These safeguards are very sensible, but less relevant to practices when they are seeking to extract their own data. In practice, this author believes that MIQUEST is a technically complex solution brought about as a response to bad historical planning and the victory of ideology over common sense.

It is also too late. Version 5, known as RFA99 (launched in October 1999, with conformant systems appearing in 2000/01), of the Rules for Accreditation of GP systems to which suppliers must conform if they wish to attract funding for GP systems, shows that MIQUEST compatibility will be a requirement.

This means that newer systems will have MIQUEST interpreters. But we have shown that they can export their data without MIQUEST. The older systems that can't will generally not have MIQUEST interpreters anyway.

This leaves me asking, who needs MIQUEST anyway? Please send answers on a postcard, or an email would do!

However, just to prove that I'm open minded and as capable of generating gobbledegook as the next anorak-wearing geek, here is a sample MIQUEST query and report. This query will provide age and sex data from a target system. Note that the report starts by reiterating the query.

Sample MIQUEST Query
Sample MIQUEST report

```
'*QRY_WDATE,19971007,07/10/1997'
'*QRY_SDATE,19971007,07/10/1997'
'*QRY_ORDER,001'
'*QRY_TITLE,AGESEX,age-sex breakdown for practice'
'*ENQ_RSPID,UNKNOWN,Unknown respondent'
'*QRY_MEDIA,D,Disk'
'*QRY_AGREE,UNKNOWN,Unknown agreement'
'*QRY_SETID,READ5AGE,Emis Read 5 standard query set - age-sex '
'*ENQ_IDENT,CHDGP,Countyshire Scheme Coordinator'
'DEFINE AGE AS @YEARS("11/05/1998",DATE_OF_BIRTH)'
ANALYSE
'GROUPED_BY SEX ("M";"F")'
'AND     AGE     ("0"-"4";"5"-"9";"10"-"14";"15"-"19";"20"-"24";"25"-
"29";"30"-"34"\'
';"35"-"39";"40"-"44";"45"-"49";"50"-"54";"55"-"59";"60"-"64";"65"-
"69";"70"\'
'-"74";"75"-"79";"80"-"84";"85"-"89";"90"-"94";"95"-"99";"100"-
"104";"105"\'
'-"109")'
```

QRY_WDATE,19971007,07/10/97

''
*QRY_SDATE,19980616,16/06/98
''*QRY_ORDER,1,
*QRY_TITLE,AGESEX,age-sex breakdown for practice
*ENQ_RSPID,NWL02,
*QRY_MEDIA,D,Disk
*QRY_AGREE,SIP,Sharing Information in Primary
*QRY_SETID,READ5AGE,Emis Read 5 standard query set - age-sex
*ENQ_IDENT,DCM,Nina Kumari
'DEFINE AGE AS @YEARS(''11/05/1998''',DATE_OF_BIRTH),
ANALYSE,,
'GROUPED_BY SEX (''M'';''F'')',,
#M is the SEX for Male,,
#F is the SEX for Female,,
'AND   AGE   (''0''-''4'';''5''-''9'';''10''-''14'';''15''-''19'';''20''-''24'';''25''-
''29'';''30''-''34'';''35''-''39'';''40''-''44'';''45''-''49'';''50''-''54'';''55''-''59'';''60''-
''64'';''65''-''69'';''70''-''74'';''75''-''79'';''80''-''84'';''85''-''89'';''90''-''94'';''95''-
''99'';''100''-''104'';''105''-''109'')',,
FROM PATIENTS,,
*RSP_IDENT,P81748,
*RSP_AUTHR,,
*RSP_RDATE,19980627,1307
&0,ANALYSE,2
SEX,AGE,
F,0-4,191
F,05-Sep,213
F,Oct-14,193
F,15-19,150
F,20-24,143
F,25-29,261
F,30-34,284
F,35-39,223
F,40-44,201
F,45-49,172
F,50-54,191
F,55-59,164
F,60-64,153
F,65-69,147

```
F,70-74,144
F,75-79,120
F,80-84,82
F,85-89,58
F,90-94,18
F,95-99,4
F,100-104,1
F,105-109,0
M,0-4,228
M,05-Sep,228
M,Oct-14,218
M,15-19,146
M,20-24,133
M,25-29,225
M,30-34,281
M,35-39,276
M,40-44,181
M,45-49,191
M,50-54,178
M,55-59,162
M,60-64,145
M,65-69,114
M,70-74,101
M,75-79,77
M,80-84,35
M,85-89,12
M,90-94,1
M,95-99,1
M,100-104,0
M,105-109,0
```

To see how this works in practice, I am indebted to Bev Ellis and her collaborators for the following description of how MIQUEST works with Vision.

MIQUEST-respondent file manager

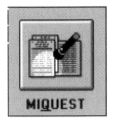

MIQUEST operates as a module accessible via a button on the main Vision module access screen.

Users of MIQUEST require appropriate authorisation via the security module, thus ensuring the security of data.

✐ Sign into Vision and access the security module by **clicking** on the Modules Menu on the front screen of Vision, then Security.

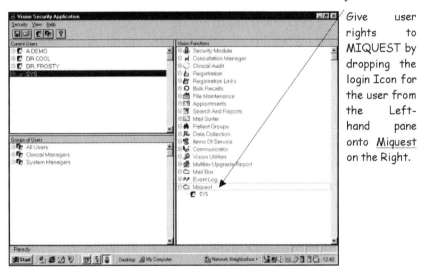

Give user rights to MIQUEST by dropping the login Icon for the user from the Left-hand pane onto Miquest on the Right.

Remember, you will have to log in again as that user for the changes to take place.

✐ **Click** the MIQUEST icon and sign on as an authorised user.

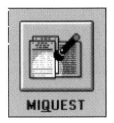

Log on to the Respondent File Manager using RFM as UserID and RFM as Password.

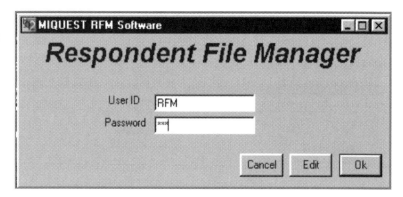

A series of tabbed forms are now available.

The Practice and Enquirer's tab must be set up before any queries can be run.

The Practice Tab

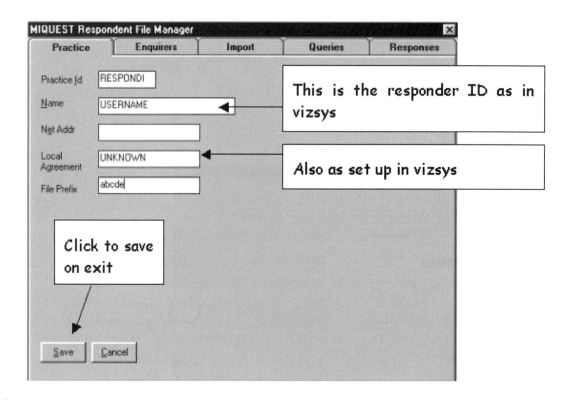

The Enquirer's Tab

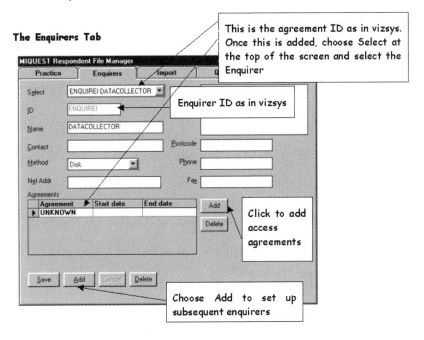

The Enquirers Tab

This is the agreement ID as in vizsys. Once this is added, choose Select at the top of the screen and select the Enquirer

Enquirer ID as in vizsys

Click to add access agreements

Choose Add to set up subsequent enquirers

The Import Tab

🖱 **Click** on the Import Tab and choose a:\.

The .hql queries will be displayed when clicking on the drive.

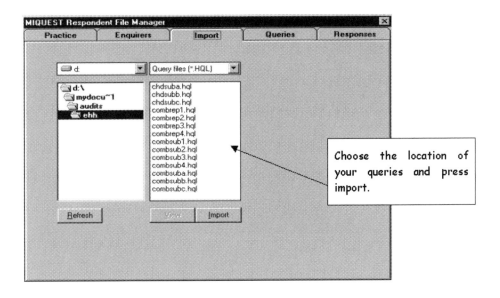

Choose the location of your queries and press import.

The Queries Tab

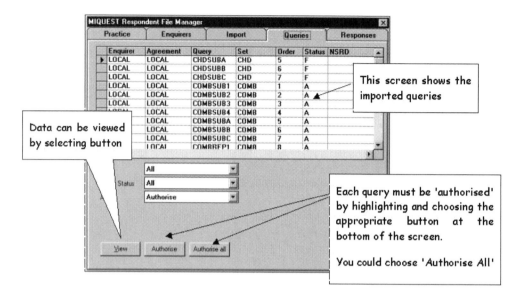

This screen shows the imported queries

Data can be viewed by selecting button

Each query must be 'authorised' by highlighting and choosing the appropriate button at the bottom of the screen.

You could choose 'Authorise All'

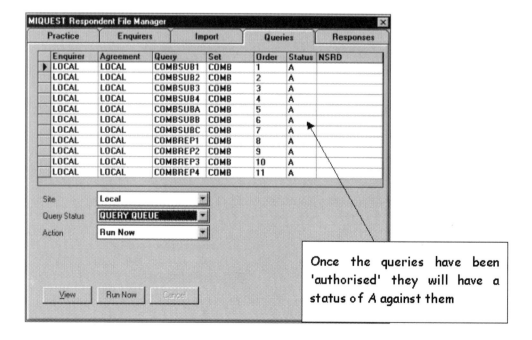

Once the queries have been 'authorised' they will have a status of A against them

The Response Tab

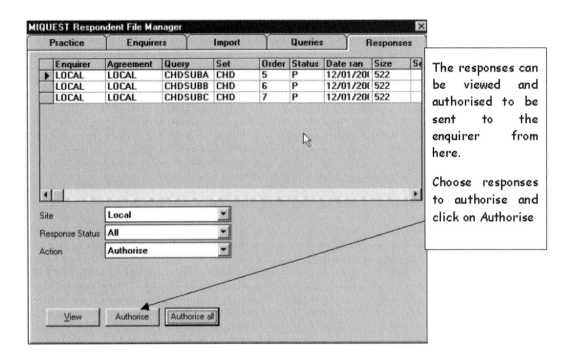

The responses can be viewed and authorised to be sent to the enquirer from here.

Choose responses to authorise and click on Authorise

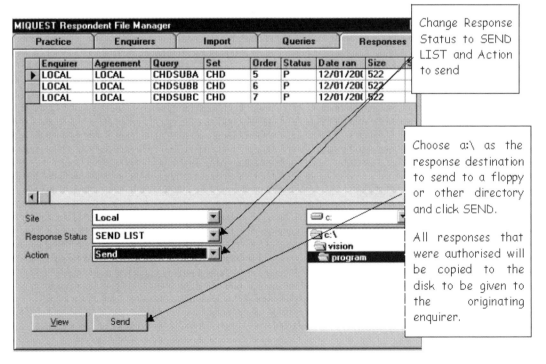

Change Response Status to SEND LIST and Action to send

Choose a:\ as the response destination to send to a floppy or other directory and click SEND.

All responses that were authorised will be copied to the disk to be given to the originating enquirer.

Index